ALLE·ZEIT·WACH
SJ
1842

Springer-Verlag France
26, rue des Carmes, 75005 Paris

J.-M. Thomassin

Otoendoscopically guided surgery

Preface by M.E. Wigand and A. Pech

with 300 figures

Springer-Verlag Paris
Berlin Heidelberg New York
London Tokyo Hong Kong
Barcelona Budapest

Professeur J.-M. Thomassin
Service de Chirurgie Cervico-maxillofaciale
C.H.R. Sainte-Marguerite
270, boulevard Sainte-Marguerite
13274 Marseille Cedex 9

ISBN 978-3-642-50965-0 ISBN 978-3-642-50963-6 (eBook)
DOI 10.1007/978-3-642-50963-6

Cover photograph: Arrangement of operating room

Dep. legal B. 19.990-1994-Edigraf-Montmeló-Barcelona
Softcover reprint of the hardcover 1st edition 1994

Contents

Abbreviations used in figures

AA	aditus ad antrum
AT	auditory tube
AEr	anterior epitympanic recess
EAC	external acoustic meatus
CC	carotid canal
Cc	chordal crest
Ct	chorda tympani nerve
Cp	cochleariform process
FC	facial canal
FG	fossula of Grivot
Fn	facial nerve
FR	facial recess
FST	supratubular fossula
H	hypotympanum
I	incus
Jb	jugular bulb
JF	jugular fossa
M	malleus
mM	manubrium of malleus
LSC	lateral semicircular canal
p	base of stapes
PC	pyramidal crest
Pe	pyramidal eminence
Pp	ponticulus promontory
Pr	promontory
Prot	protympanum
PS	posterior sinus
PTS	posterior tympanic sinus
Ptc	posterior tympanic crest
OW	oval window
RW	round window
s	stapes
scTm	semi-canal for tensor tympani muscle
SE	styloid eminence
Sp	subiculum promontory
ST	sinus tympani
St	stapedius tendon
STP	posterior sinus tympani (Proctor)
TA	tympanic antrum
Tn	tympanic nerve (Jacobson)
TS	tympanic sinus
tt	tegmen tympani
Ttm	tensor tympani muscle

Preface

The endoscope with magnifying lens systems and angled view has, in all oto-rhino-laryngology, been developed from a basically diagnostical tool into a surgical instrument. Earlier, it served to see what exists. Nowadays, it is continuously changing what one does.

Jean-Marc Thomassin's book "Otoendoscopically guided surgey" appears as the first guide into this new field of otoendoscopic control of microsurgery of the ear. The author has achieved to compile and codify what, during recent years, was already looked at by him and by a "happy few" of otological pilots. But, he has also added new insights into this matter. One may say that he has provided a solid basis for both the scholars and the experts who want to enrich their arsenal of otosurgical techniques.

Who was privileged, as I have been, to follow Professor Thomassin's work over a couple of years while observing his masterpieces of otophotography at conferences and workshops must attest him a second mastership, namely the composition of an artful manual of this new approach to tympanoplasty. Middle ear operations, modified by the closest inspection of the surgical field perceivable at present, that is the postulate of this book. A challenge and a promise at the same time.

If one looks closer at his concepts, one will find three major chapters, among shorter paragraphs on history, instrumentation, anesthesia and results, dealing with 1) endoscopic anatomy of the middle ear cavities, 2) otoscopic pathological findings, and 3) cholesteatoma surgery in all its variations. Otoendoscopic surgery for other indications like congenital malformations, injuries or benign tumours, is logically implemented but with shorter instructions.

The advantages of otoendoscopy have become obvious: the basic training of residents will be enriched by the possibility of becoming familiar with the variations of difficult to understand epi-, pro- and retrotympanic sub-regions. During microsurgical procedures, the recognition of pathologic changes in niches, recesses or occluded tunnels is considerably facilitated. The disadvantages of the operating microscope —reduced brightness and bad focus with higher magnifieations, no angled view— can be compensated by additional endoscopy with the instrument's tip close to the target and with the view "around the corner".

While thus visualizing remote areas or hidden spots by a rigid magnifying endoscope with an angled view direction apparently no patho-anatomical secret remains undiscovered. What can be inspected can be cleaned, there are adequate instruments. This fact makes the analysis of surgical failures more plausible.

As Thomassin in this book also illustrates, the second look or revision operations can be realized more effectively and less aggressively by utilizing the endoscope via a minimal retroauricular cutaneous approach. C. Jansen had imaginated this method for adults in the seventies. The reoperation of individual cases apparently can be enhanced by this technique. Endoscopy as the key for a "monitored microsurgery" like for the "non-aggressive revision operation", that is the message I have learned from Jean-Marc Thomassin.

One may be curious for future comprehension of rules deciding on success or failure of certain methods by detecting their either surgical or biological reasons with help of this optical tool. In so far, what is called monitoring may reveal itself as a multiplier of microsurgical skill.

I believe, therefore, that this beautiful book should reach every otologist devoted to the art of functional plastic surgery of the ear.

Professor M.E. Wigand

Preface

This book by Professor Jean-Marc Thomassin bears witness to the present change of direction in the surgery of the middle ear. For 40 years the operating microscope has allowed decisive progress, but its use has been hampered by the existence of inevitable blind spaces in the auricular cavities. Yet these hidden zones, inacessible to deliberate surgery under visual monitoring, are very important since 15 % of cholesteatomas are situated here. Endoscopic guided surgery permits such monitoring, thanks to the use of appropriate lens systems, but calls for the acquisition of perfectly integrated techniques by the otologist to obtain the desired results. The codification of these techniques is the subject of this book. It is based on a major anatomic study. Remarkable photographs of dissections of 50 petrous bones perfectly complement our theoretic knowledge of the retrotympanum and supply an important concept: that 60% of tympanic sinuses exhibit a narrow orifice which makes surgical exploration difficult, the more so since they may be prolonged as a subfacial recess. The necessary equipment is specified in its smallest details: optical systems of 2,7 mm diameter and 30 to 70 degrees of angle, the support necessary to tree both of surgeon's hands, angled micro-instruments : suckers, hooks and dissectors.

The indications for endoscopic guided surgery currently seem very wide. Monitoring of ossiculoplasties, the search for perilymphatic fistulas, and the treatment of certain retraction pockets may all benefit from it. However, cholesteoma certainly represents its main field of application: mastoidectomy, antro-atticotomy, the fashioning of a posterior tympanotomy, are still performed under the microscope, though this is replaced by lens systems for the difficult zones of the epitympanum and the supratubal fossa and, especially, the retrotympanum. Revision procedures after closed techniques remain indispensable. Despite this progress, it is only rarely possible to dispense with modern imaging. It can detect residual cholesteatomas of 3 mm diameter, but the cavities of the middle ear must be free and aerated, and this condition is satisfied in only 30% of cases. Endoscopic guided surgery using a retroauricular and/or a transmeatal approach considerably reduces the severity of these reoperations and may even allow the patients to be operated as days cases. Revision of the operative cavities appears reliable, and the eradication of cholesteatoma pearls is possible. It certainly represents the method of the future.

This manual is intended to be essentially practical. It does not conceal the difficulties. The management of the optical sytems is not a simple matter: the 70 degree angle lens systems are tricky to use and must be reserved for the hidden regions; the surgeon must familiarise himself with the new territories it reveals, and it is important for him to use it in every tympanoplasty if he is familiarise himself with its employment. Nor is the surgical technique any simpler, it calls for the acquisition of a new operative procedure. Therefore, the different stages of the various operations are set out very clearly.

This work, whose style is sober and concise, contains some remarkable illustrations -otoscopic, anatomic, and especially surgical, constituting a true photographic record of the operative stages. It well reflects the exceptional qualities of Professor Jean-Marc Thomassin: the seriousness of his study, his sense of innovation, the basic care for progress in surgical practice which remains one of his fundamental passions. he Has written a real manual of this new form of otologic surgery, which I am certain, is detined to have a great future.

Professor A. Pech

Acknowledgments

This book is the outcome of ten years' work which has allowed me to developp this new technique in aural surgery, years that have provided me with much pleasure and great satisfaction.

The project of setting down on paper, classifying and communicating this new video-assisted surgical procedure was also great, but complex. None of it would have been possible without the goodwill and collaboration of all concerned.

I have therefore to thank here the entire medical theam that has worked with me from the first steps in this research up to the applications we employ today.

The development of a specific form of anesthesia for this surgery has been the work of a team of anesthetists : Drs. J. Conciatori, C Rud and P Vilcoq. I am also indebted to the nursing and equipment staff, especially to Madame Schaller-Verihle for her patience beside me during these various procedures, which have required methodical research for the exploitation of the imaging techniques.

I am also particularly grateful to my close collaborators : JM Inedjian and DS Korchia, and to JM Duchon-Doris, who, through his research work, has greatly facilitated the documentation related to the chapter on endoscopic anatomy.

To all of these I express my sincere thanks for their collaboration and their patience.

Particular acknowledgments

I am deeply indebted for the achievement of these studies to the active collaboration of the Karl Storz laboratories. They have provided all the supporting equipment needed for the diffusion and development of video-assisted endoscopic guided surgery. I therefore express my thanks to Madame Sybill-Storz-Relling, who understood at an early stage the importance of this new otologic technique.

Finally, I would like to dedicate this book to my very dear friend, Brigitte Rouze. Her love and skill throughout the preparation of this book have allowed me to form contacts, and to ensure collaboration, with the Karl Storz Laboratories for the construction of the endoscopes. International diffusion has also been her responsibility. She has furthermore taken an active part in the editing of this manual.

History

From the outset, endoscopic investigation of the tympanic membrane was hampered by difficulties of illumination. In the 17th century Borel used a concave mirror to reflect sunlight and was thus able to proceed to cursory examination of the external acoustic meatus and also of the tympanic membrane. In the middle of the 19th century Toynbee for the first time focussed a candle flame as a light source for an otoscope fitted with a reflecting mirror. However, no real development of otoscopic instruments could take place until the arrival of the electric light. It was only the introduction of the binocular lens with several magnifications that ushered otoscopy and the surgery of deafness into its modern period.

Hopkins (1966) developed a system of optical rods that allowed the construction of rigid endoscopic tubes. The technical quality of the lenses, lit from cold light sources, allowed very simple, rapid and precise otoendoscopic examination of the tympanum. Having arrived at this stage of investigation of the tympanic membrane, it remained to take a decisive step (ie)? the peroperative use of the system to visualise the middle ear cavities. The operating microscope gave global vision of all the cavities of the middle ear, except for the retrotympanic region of the main cavity. Jako (1966) and Zini (1967) (fig. 1) conceived the use of stainless steel micro-mirrors to investigate the sinus tympani. This system, reflecting the light of the operating microscope, was useful in experienced hands but was not reliable for the eradication of (epidermal) lesions at this site.

Mer (1967) employed a flexible fiberscope to examine the middle ear cavity. Marquet (1974) introduced an endoscope 1.7 mm in diameter through a tympanic perforation to observe the tympanic cavity. He already foresaw the great possibilities of this technique and wrote: "the retrotympanic regions, such as the sinus tympani, can be observed in a precise manner."

Nomura (1982) developed a new system of rigid endoscopy which he called the "needle otoscope". At its distal end a prism refracted the light through an angle of 90°. He used this for the diagnosis of lesions of the tympanic cavity at operation. Kanzaki (1983) was the first to anticipate the importance of endoscopy in postoperative surveillance of the posterior cavities of the middle ear in patients operated for cholesteaoma by a closed technique. Under local anesthesia, he introduced an endoscope via a retroauricular incision and reported a series of 26 cases.

Wullstein (1984) had a micrometric system manufactured by the firm of Storz: the ototympanoscope. Using two endoscopes, and under visual control, this allowed the passage through a perforation of an endoscope 2.7 mm in diameter and with 30° and 70° angles of vision. The disadvantage of this endoscope was that both hands of the surgeon were engaged, thus preventing any treatment procedure. Ultimately, it found little general use.

Bluestone (1986) demonstrated the value of Nomura's endoscope for examination of retraction pockets, as well as their extension to the posterior wall of the tympanic cavity in children. Jansen (1985) used fine optical systems for operative monitoring of the

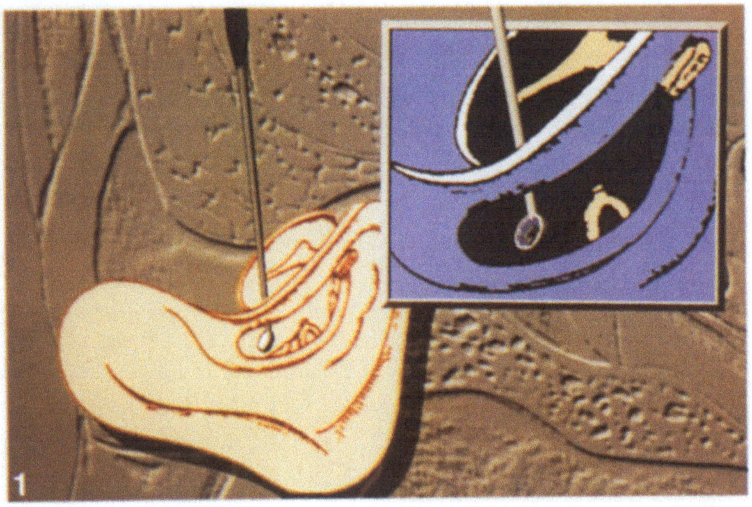

Fig. 1. Indirect microtympanoscopy by means of micro-mirrors

middle ear cavities. Martin (1989) used systems with 0° and 30° angles for survey of retraction pockets in adults.

In 1984 we began to practice peroperative monitoring of the posterior recesses of the tympanic cavity using a 2.7 mm optical system with a 70° angle (Storz) as used for Wullstein's ototympanoscope. In 1985 we performed endoscopic surgery of the sinus tympani (fig. 2 a,b). From 1988 we developed video-monitored endoscopic guided surgery for the retrotympanum and anterior epitympanum by coupling the endoscope to a microcamera. In 1990 we carried out a second monitoring stage for cholesteatomas operated by tympanoplasty, using a closed technique with a minimal cutaneous approach in the retroauricular region. In over 700 of cases this surgical procedure was very often combined with survey of the tympanic cavity, more especially of the retrotympoanum, via a limited transmeatal route.

With the same aim of allowing monitoring of the cavities of the middle ear, the tubotympanic microfiberoscopy developed by Yamashita (1980), Jansen (1985), Kimura (1989) and introduced into France by Magnan (1990) may constitute a useful alternative. However, at present the quality of the images is not as satisfactory with these fibers of 0.9 to 1.4 mm diameter as those obtained with rigid optical systems. Moreover, the absence of distal support does not allow survey of the entire tympanic cavity or epitympanum. However, this technique has provided valuable information on the state of the tubal mucosa in otitic disease.

References

Bremond G, Magnan J, Chays A, De Gasquet R (1990) Endoscopie de la trompe d'Eustache. Ann Otol Laryngol (Paris) 107 : 15-19

Eichner H (1978) Eline Mother and Baby-scope-optic zur trommelfelle un Mittelohr-Endoskopie. Laryngol Rhinol Otol (Stuttg) 57 : 872-876

Gonzalez C, Bluestone C (1986) Visualization of a retraction pocket cholesteatoma : indications for use of the middle ear telescope in children. Laryngoscope 96 : 109-110

Hopkins H (1976) Optical principles of the endoscope. In : Berci G (Ed) Endoscopy. New York, Appleton, Century crafts, p 3

Jako G (1966) The posterior bony ear canal wall and the antrum threshold angle in conservative middle ear surgery. Laryngoscope 76 : 1260-1271

Jansen C (1985) Endoscopy and surgery of the eustachian tube. Politzer Society Conference, Montreux, Switzerland, september 4-8, 1985

Jansen C (1991) Rigid and flexible endoscopy of the middle ear and the eustachian tube. Politzer Society Conference on the reality in ear surgery and otoneursurgery, Maastricht, Netherlands, june 16-21, 1991

Kanzaki J (1983) Postoperative aural attico-antroscopy for cholesteatoma. ORL 45 : 290-296

Kimura Y, Yamaguchi H, Cheng S (1989) Direct observation of the tympanic cavity by superfine fiberscope. Nippon Jibiinkoka Gakkai Kaiko 92 : 233-238

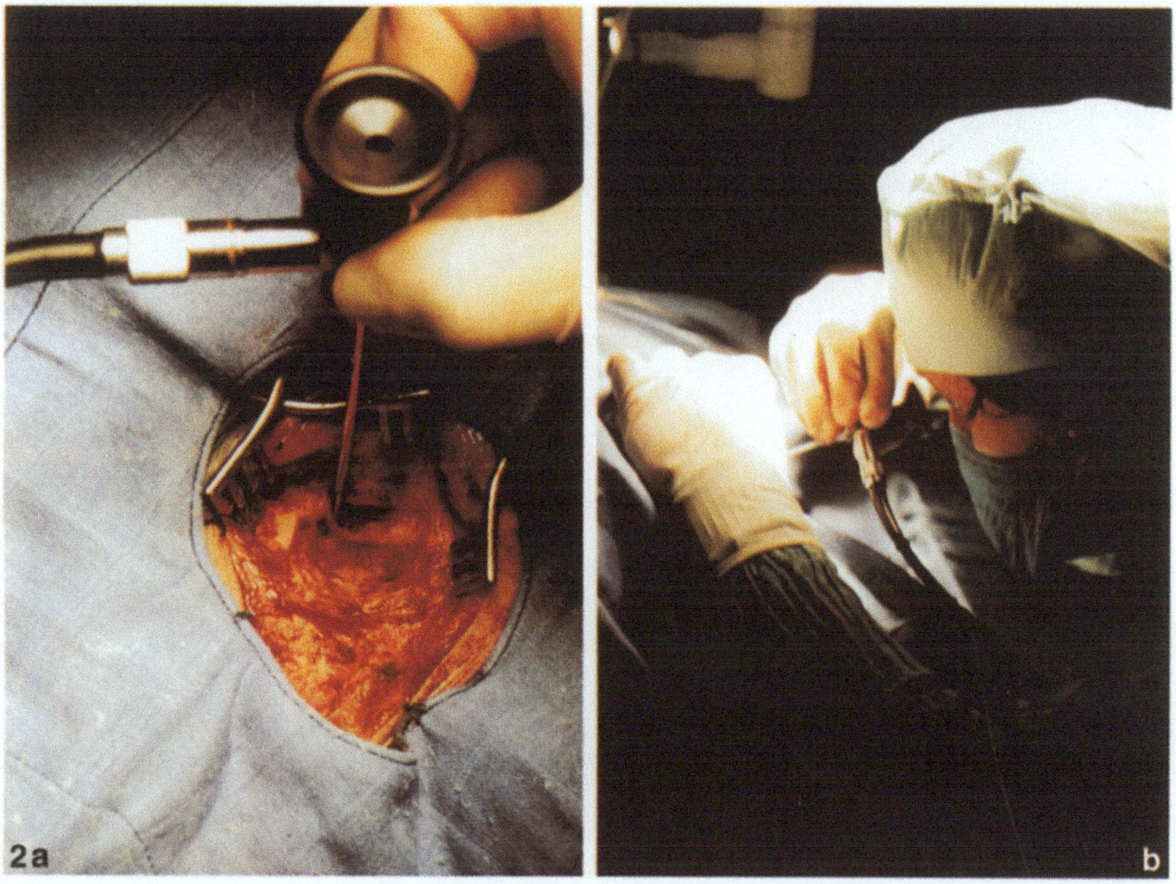

Fig. 2 a, b. Peroperative survey of posterior region of tympanic cavity (1984) using Wullstein's optical system, 2.7 mm diameter, 70° angle

Mer S, Derbysthire A, Brushenko A (1967) Fiberoptic endotoscopes for examining the middle ear. Arch Otolaryngol 85 : 387-393

Nomura Y (1982) A needle otoscope (an instrument of endotoscopy of the middle ear). Acta Otolaryngol (Stockh) 93 : 73-79

Poe D, Rebeiz E, Panknatov M, Shapshory S (1992) Transtympanic endoscopy of the middle ear. Laryngoscope 102 : 993-996

Thomassin JM, Duchon-Doris JM, Emram B, Rud C, Conciatori J, Vilcoq P (1990) Otochirurgie endoscopique premier bilan. Ann Otol Laryngol (Paris) 107 : 564-570

Willemot J, Marquet J, Van Clooster R, Seddee G, Segal S (1975) Les techniques d'endoscopie et de reproduction de l'image en otorhinolaryngologie. Acta Otorhinolaryngol Belg 29 : 299-316

Wullstein H, Wullstein S (1986) Tympanoplastik osteoplastiche Epitympanotomie. Thieme-Verlag, Stuttgart, New York

Yamashita K (1980) Endoscopic testing method of eustachian tube. Ann Otol Rhinol Laryngol 89 (suppl 68)

Zini C (1967) La microtympanoscopie indirecte. Rev Laryngol Otol Rhinol (Bord) 88 : 736-738

Endoscopic anatomy of the middle ear cavities

Training in endoscopic anatomy using an optical axis is an essential preliminary to surgery under video monitoring. Unlike the books of descriptive anatomy,. the surgeon working with an oblique angle endoscope must convey a three-dimensional image, which will allow him to know exactly where he is. We have chosen to describe the endoscopic anatomy of certain regions of the middle ear cavity in terms of optical systems with different angles of vision, ie 0°, 30° and 70°. These regions, which are difficult of access or impossible to see with the operating microscope, may become so thanks to endoscopy.

Retrotympanic region of the tympanic cavity

Descriptive anatomy

In classical descriptive anatomy the posterior wall of the tympanic cavity is represented as an approximately vertical groove open forward and inward, a gap into the tympanic embedded between the tympanic wall and the labyrinthine wall (fig. 3).

Its anatomic complexity is due to the many prominences and depressions present on its surface, and also to their numerous variations. Guerrier and Andréa (1976) have proposed a systematisation of this region around a central feature that is always identifiable: the pyramidal eminence (fig. 4). This is the point of convergence of a series of five bony prominences:

– laterally and transversely: the chordal ridge

– below and longitudinally: the pyramidal ridge

– medially and transversely: two ridges, one situated in front, the ponticulus, and one behind, the posterior tympanic ridge.

– above and oblique outward: the prominence of the bend of the facial canal.

On the basis of these five prominences, four regions may be defined;

– between the chordal and pyramidal ridges: the fossula of Grivot (posterior or facial sinus)

– between the pyramidal ridge and the ponticulus: the sinus tympani

– between the ponticulus and the facial canal: the posterior tympanic sinus of Proctor

– between the facial canal and the chordal ridge: the facial recess.

The region of the sinus tympani can only be visualised by the use of an oblique optical system angled between 50° and 70°, since the axis of the former is perceptibly at right angles to the axis of the external acoustic meatus.

Endoscopic anatomy

With a 70° lens system the circle of vision includes the following anatomic environment: for the right ear, the prominence of the promontory is recognised above, the head of the stapes is seen vanishing laterally, while behind there is a constant feature which forms a real landmark in video-monitored surgery: the pyramidal eminence and the stapedius tendon (fig. 5 a-d).

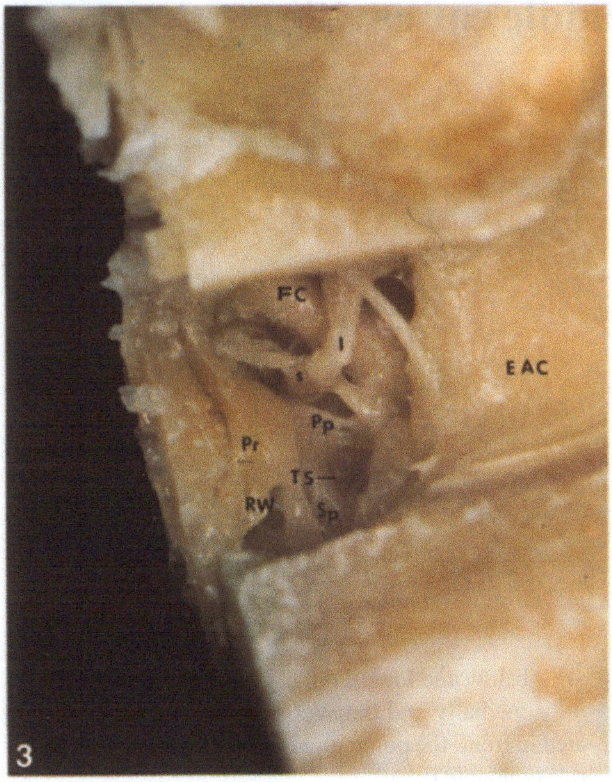

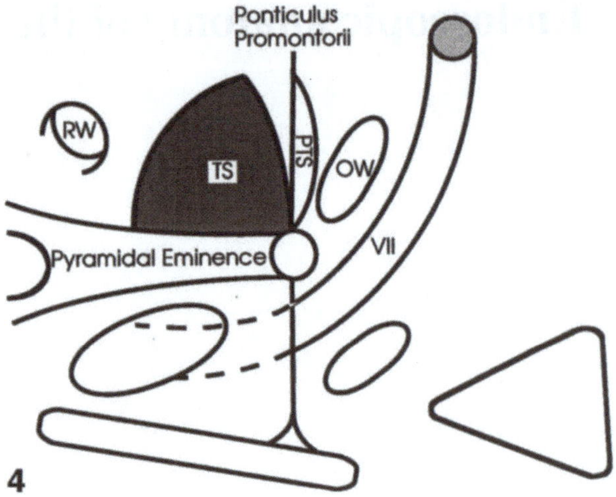

4

Fig. 3. Dissection of a left petrous: view of retrotympanum and sinus tympani

Fig. 4. Orientation of posterior region of tympanic cavity (Guerrier, Andréa) (left ear)

Sinus tympani

Circular movement of the endoscope will reveal the orifice of the sinus tympani. This is usually perceived as elliptical in shape with the main axis longitudinal, slightly oblique upward and inward, measuring between 2.5 and 3.5 mm in length, and the lesser axis of 1 to 2 mm. It is demarcated by two bony ridges: the ponticulus above and the subiculum promontori below (fig. 6). Its depth is very variable, being given by Donaldson (1970) as 2.93 mm, by Saito (1971) as 3.75 mm, and by Guerrier (1976) as 2 to 3 mm.

It seems inadequate to base a classification solely on criteria of size (depth, diameter). Therefore we have decided to classify the tympanic sinuses in terms of their accessibility to surgical exploration, and have grouped them into three types (based on an endoscopic study of 50 right and left temporal bones).

Access to the sinus tympani is easy

Shallow sinuses with shelving margins constituted 20% of our cases (fig. 7 a-d). At endoscopy, they appear as simple depressions rather than cavities proper. Their boundaries are ill-defined, especially below, where in 25% of cases the subiculum is either absent or poorly developed. There is a continuity between the sinus tympani and the cells of the protympanum. The subiculum may also sometimes present as a bony bridge stretching between the styloid eminence and the promontory.

Access to the sinus tympani is difficult

This was the case in 60% of our series. There is a deep depression, with well-defined margins and a narrow entry orifice (fig. 8 a-f), whose diameter is less than that of the rest of the cavity. Although the walls are always smooth, without any roughness or small cells, the blind curettage of such a cavity is bound to be incomplete and the source of residual pathology. Hence the opportunity (and the necessity) for video-monitored endoscopic surgery.

Some 12% of these forms exhibit a posterosuperior prolongation, a sort of actual invagination beneath the pyramidal eminence and the faclal canal (fig. 8 f). Even in these very deep cases the use of an endoscope

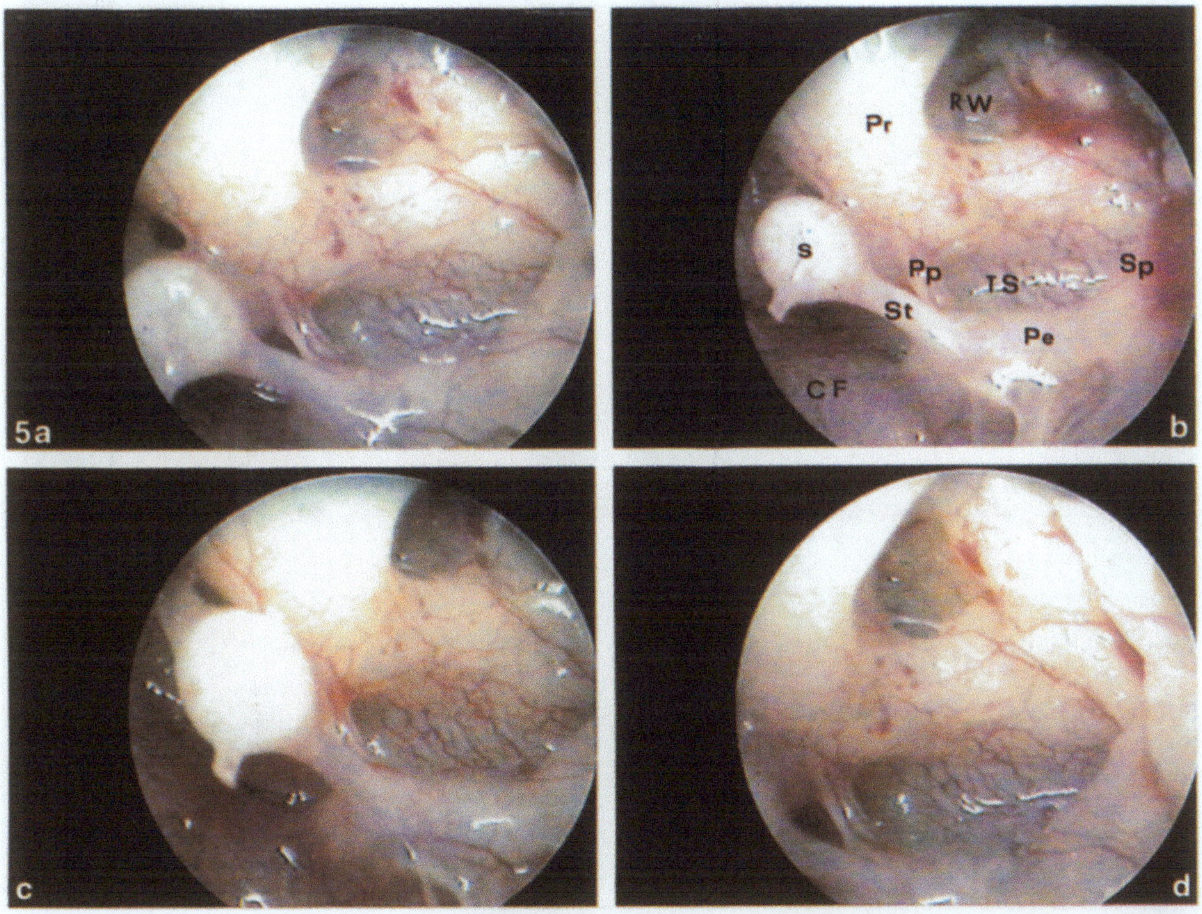

Fig. 5 a-d. Right ear: retrotympanic region. Endoscopic view of retrotympanum with 70° angle, 2.7 mm diameter, optical system. **a-c** Sinus tympani; **d** entry orifice of sinus tympani

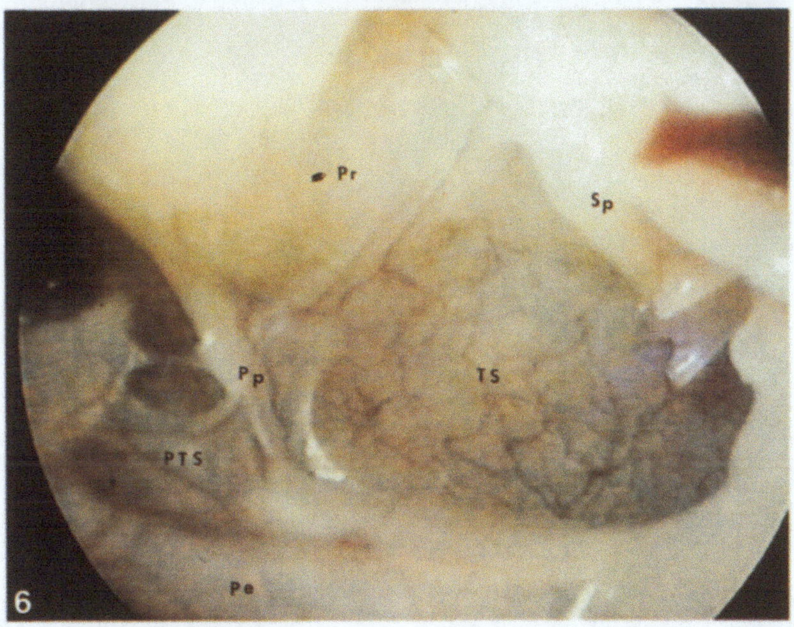

Fig. 6. Right ear: orifice of sinus tympani

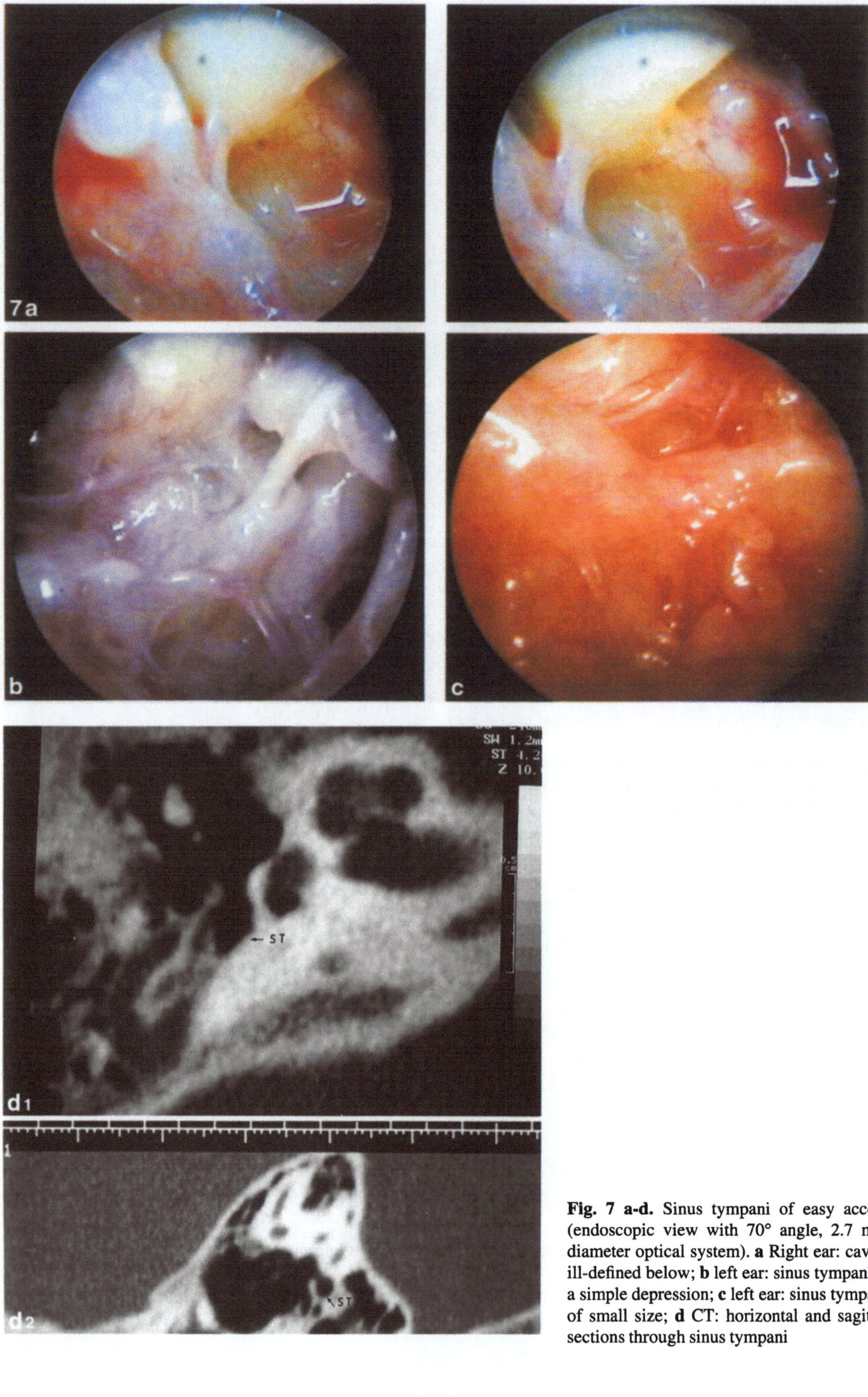

Fig. 7 a-d. Sinus tympani of easy access (endoscopic view with 70° angle, 2.7 mm diameter optical system). **a** Right ear: cavity ill-defined below; **b** left ear: sinus tympani is a simple depression; **c** left ear: sinus tympani of small size; **d** CT: horizontal and sagittal sections through sinus tympani

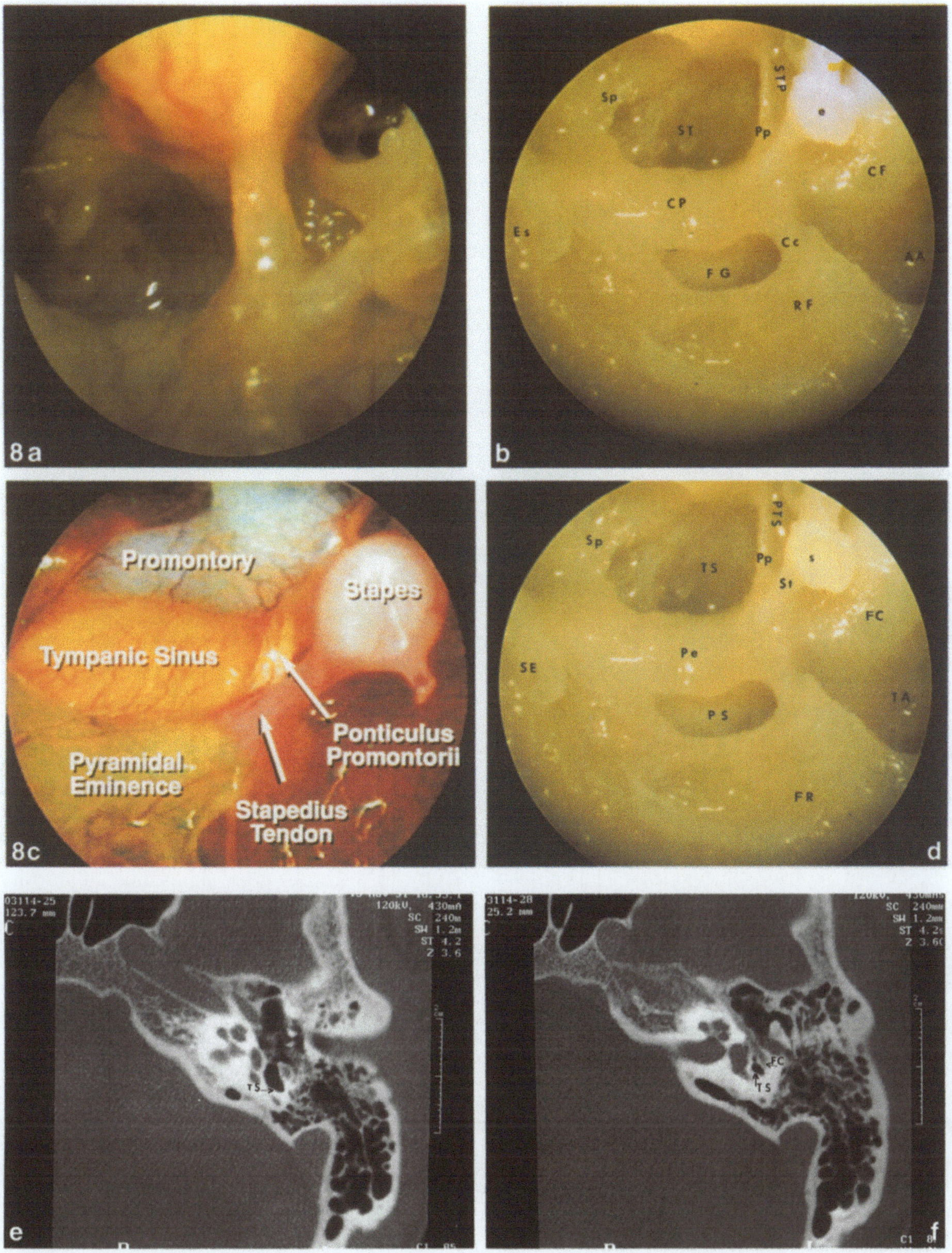

Fig. 8 a-f. Sinus tympani of difficult access (endoscopic view with 70° angle, 2.7 mm diameter optical system). **a** Left ear: deep cavity with well-defined margins, ponticulus very thick; **b** left ear: larger orifice with posterosuperior subfacial prolongation; **c** left ear: entry orifice narrowed to lesser diameter than cavity; **d** left ear: narrow deep cavity; **e, f** CT, horizontal section. In this case there is a posterosuperior prolongation under the facial canal

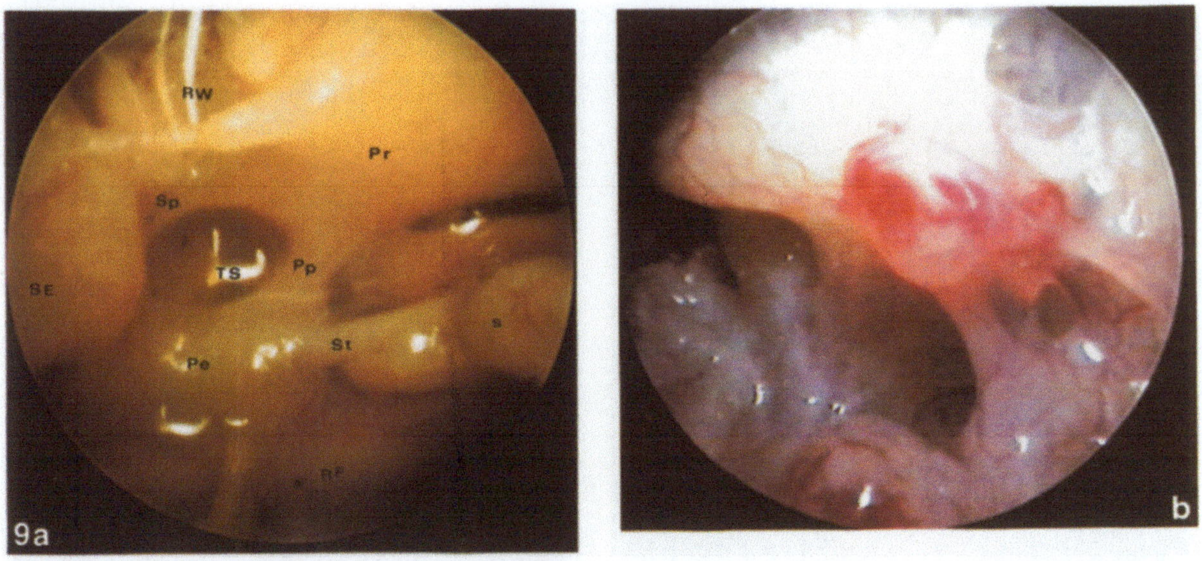

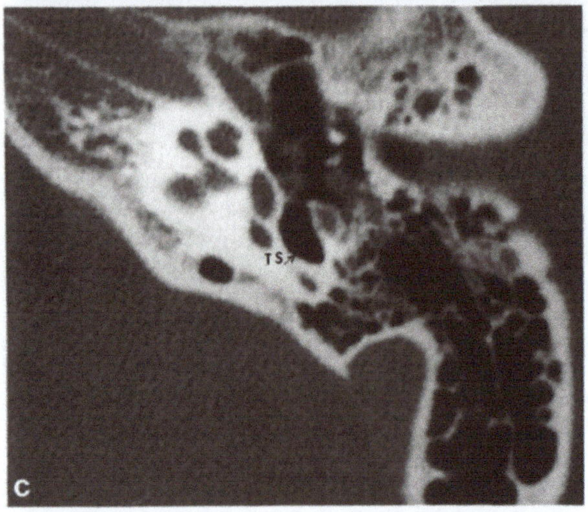

Fig. 9 a-c. Intermediate sinus tympani (endoscopic view with 70° angle, 2.7 mm diameter optical system). **a** Left ear: deep cavity with shelving margins; **b** left ear: deep cavity with absent subiculum; **c** CT, horizontal section through sinus tympani: deep cavity, wide entry orifice

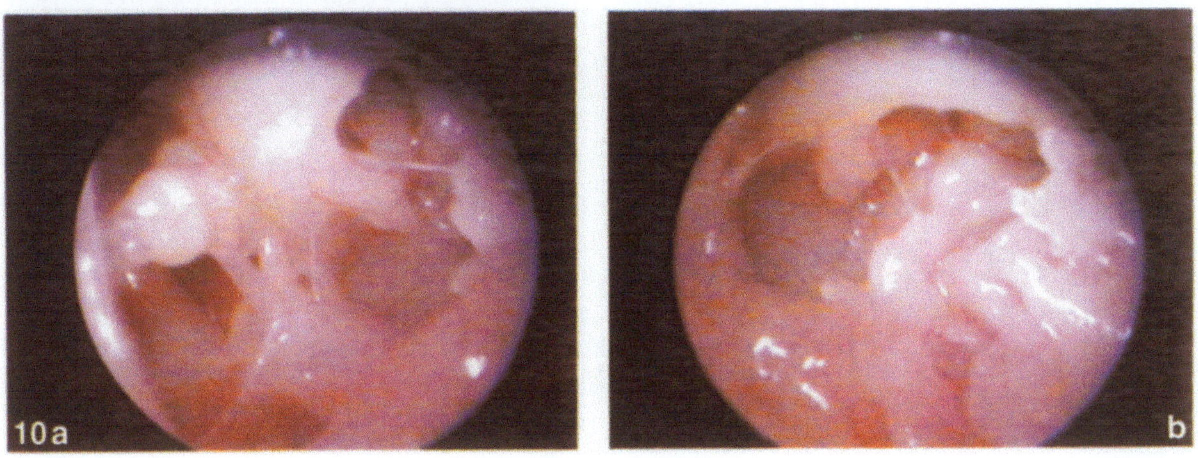

Fig. 10 a, b. Sinus tympani (endoscopic view with 70° angle, 2.7 mm diameter optical system). **a** Right ear: global view of retrotympanum; **b** prominence of styloid eminence, partly concealing round recess

with a 70° visual angle allows complete surveillance of the entire cavity.

Intermediate cases (fig. 9 a-c)

There were 20% of tympanic sinuses that could not be classified in one or other of the two preceding categories. The cavity was certainly deep, but its orifice of entry was wide with shelving margins and there was no posterior prolongation.

Styloid eminence

Usually this prominence is not very evident. It is practically always identifiable at the floor of the tympanic cavity, but in 10% of cases we found a very developed styloid eminence forming a prominence within the tympanic cavity (fig. 10 a,b) and possibly even narrowing the entry to the orifice of the sinus tympani.

This study of the endoscopic anatomy leads to the following conclusions:

– despite the wide variety of shapes and dimensions of the various fossulae of the retro-tympanum, endoscopy has made it possible to explore the smallest recesses without any blind zone, just as at microscopic observation. This new possibility is particularly evident in the 60% of cases where acess to the sinus tympani is difficult. Although, in some ears, an optical system of 30° angle and 2.7 mm diameter allows visualisation of the posterior region of the tympanum, usually only a 2.7 mm system of 70° angle permits surveillance of the base of the entire cavity of the sinus tympani. The lytic action of a cholesteatoma tends to create a hollow medial and posterior to this depression.

– There is also a symmetry of anomalies between the right and left sides in the same dissection specimen, whether the ponticulus is incomplete, the sinus tympani deep or shallow. Therefore it is important, in cases of bilateral cholesteatomatous pathology, to make a careful note of the anatomic features in the operative protocol.

– When there is prolapse of the jugular bulb, this makes the sinus tympani even deeper (fig. 11 a-d). Despite this difficulty, the proper choice of optical system allows perfect surveillance of every recess of the posterior wall of the tympanic cavity.

The protympanum

This constitutes the bony portion of the auditory tube, and appears through the endoscope with a 0° system in the shape of a funnel with an elliptical orifice 5 mm high by 3 mm (fig. 12a-d). It is overhung by the semi canal of the tensor tympani muscle. Like the wall of the main tympanic cavity, it is covered by a single and identical mucosa. It measures 10 to 14 mm in length. Its medial wall is formed by the lateral wall of the carotid canal (fig. 13 a-d) and is very thin. Therefore, in certain extensive cholesteatomas careful attention must be given to ablation of the epidermal matrix on this wall since the internal carotid may be exposed.

The hypoptympanum

Here, the morphology is quite simple. It corresponds to the inferior or jugular wall, also known as the hypotympanic recess, situated below the external auditory meatus. In 70% of cases, according to Proctor (1963), the presence of the bulb of the jugular vein produces a dome beneath the floor which may sometimes project very far upwards into the tympanic cavity (fig. 14 a,b). Viewing with a 30° optical system improves the image of the deep parts. Likewise, its circular movement allows inclusion of the following anatomic setting: the posterior part of the tympanic floor, the styloid protuberance of Politzer, the superior orifice of the tympanic canal transmitting the tympanic nerve (of Jacobson), and finally a very irregular zone pitted with cellular cavities which corresponds to the sublabyrinthine and anticochlear pathways (fig. 15 a-d).

Certain extensions of cholesteatoma to this region require the surgeon to burr the cellular bone in order to clear out this recess properly. The step down below the plane of the inferior wall of the external auditory meatus constitutes a hindrance to viewing of this site under the operating microscope. The use of optical rods allows more precise monitoring with the aim of eradication of a cholesteatoma of this recess.

The anterior epitympanum

This corresponds to the free preossicular space (head of the malleus). The anterior part of the epitympanic cavity, which is difficult to view under the operating microscope even after ablation of the head of the malleus, is extended in almost every case —96% according to Andréa (1976)— by an orifice giving acess to a

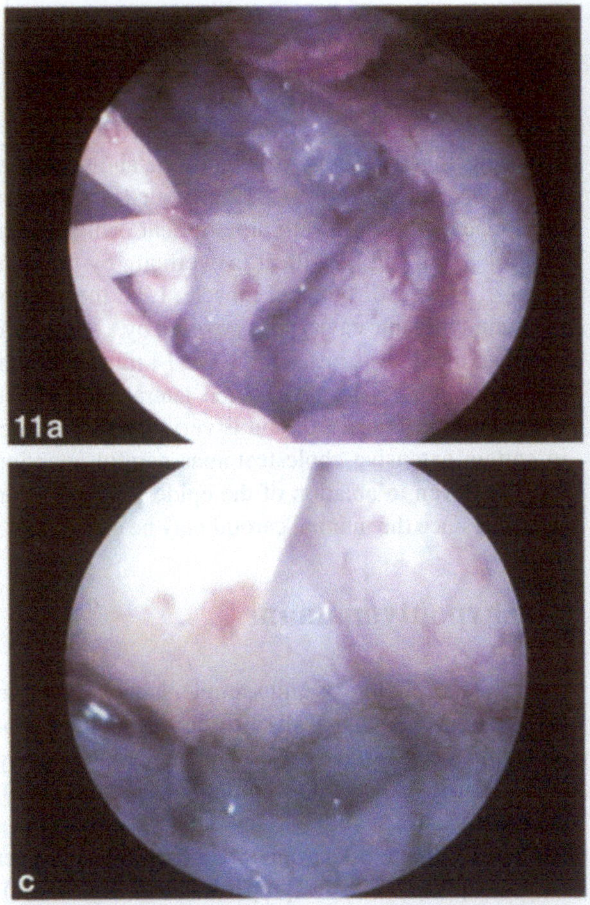
11a
b
c
d

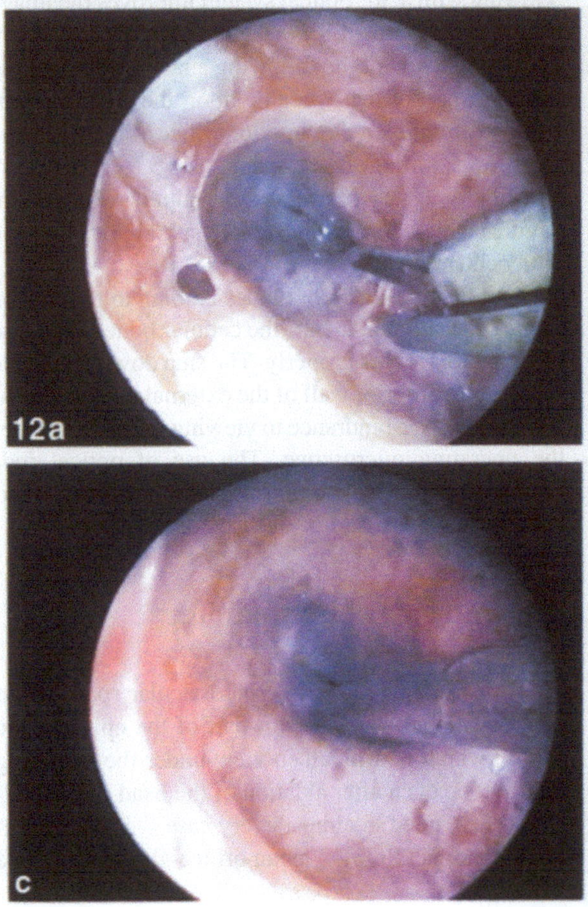
12a
b
c
d

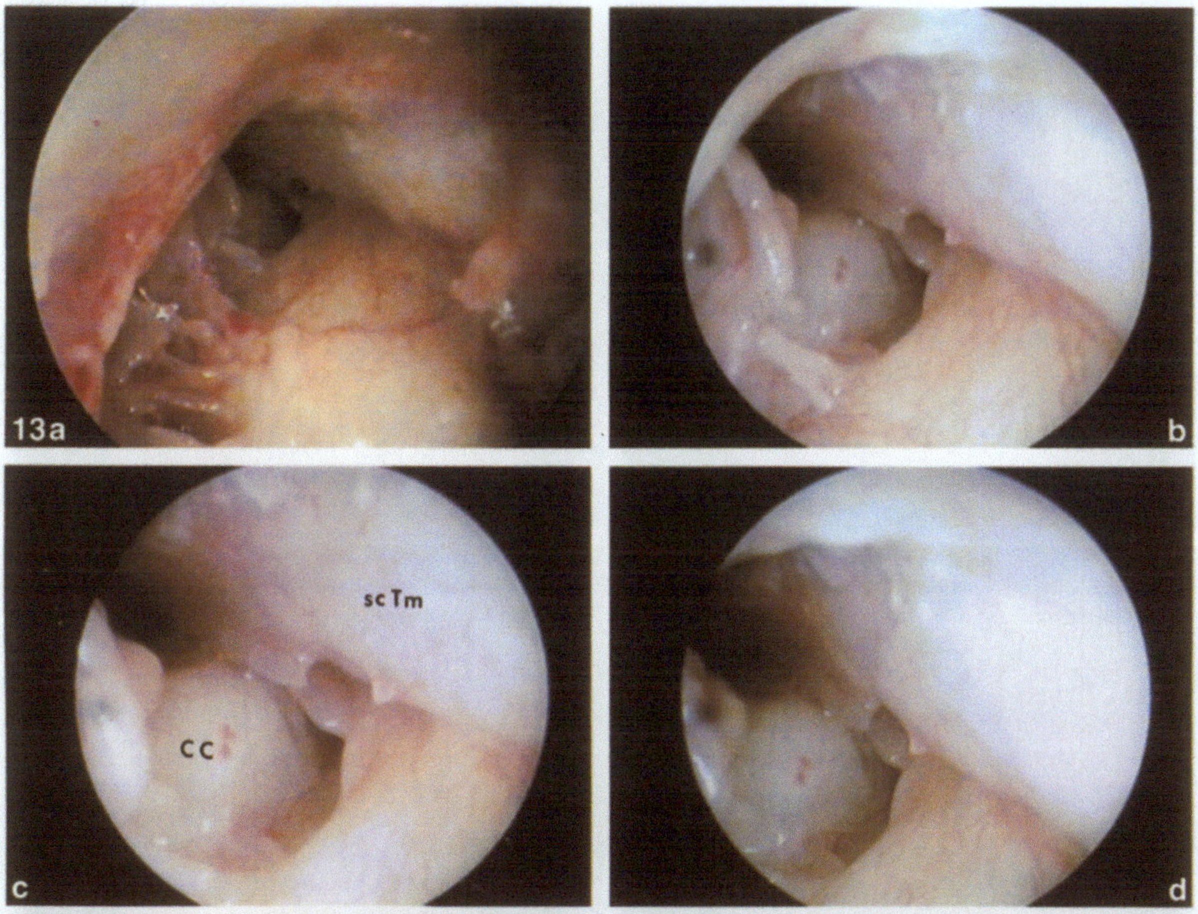

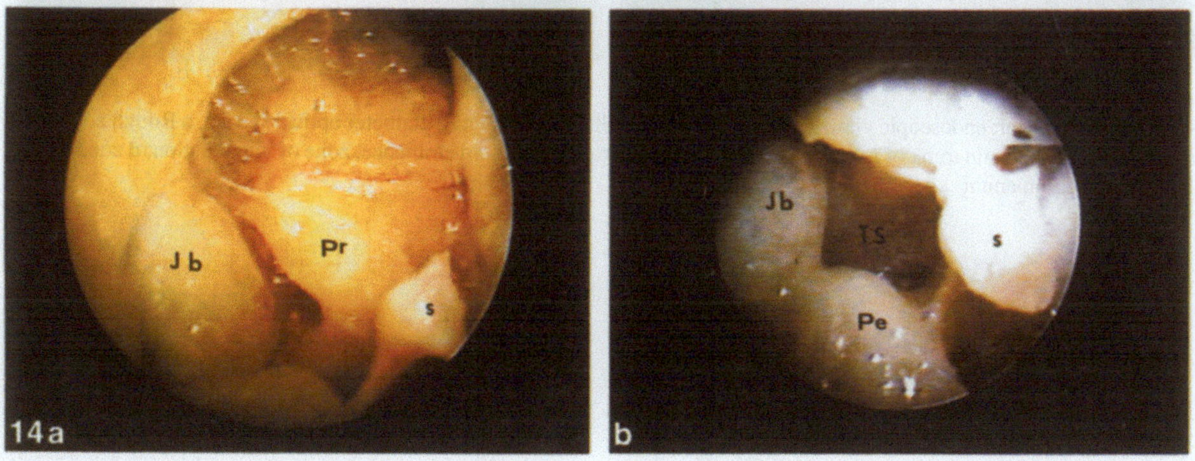

Fig. 13 a-d. Left ear: region of protympanum (optical system 0° angle, 2.7 mm diameter). **a** View of tympanic cavity; **b-d** prominence of carotid canal and canal of tensor tympani muscle

Fig. 14 a, b. Right ear: jugular dome (anatomic specimen). **a** View of tympanic cavity; **b** appearance with 70° optical system showing prominence of jugular dome and of styloid eminence

←

Fig. 11 a-d. Right ear: endoscopic view of tympanic cavity. **a** View with 0° angle optical system. Bulge of jugular dome; **b-d** view with 70° angle optical system. The sinus tympani appears to have more depth because of the high position of the jugular dome

Fig. 12 a-d. Right ear: protympanum, orifice of auditory tube (0° optical system). **a-c** Funnel-shaped protympanum; **d** tubal isthmus

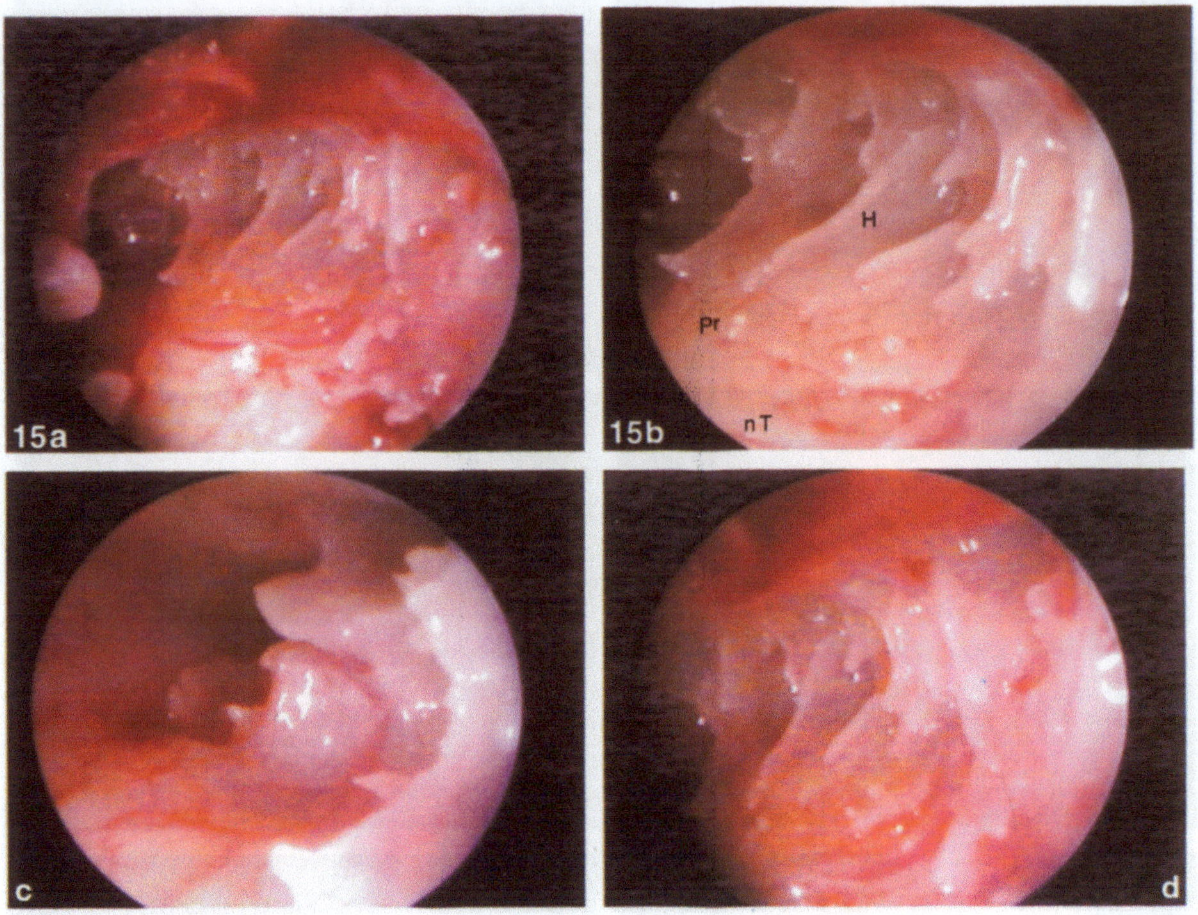

Fig. 15 a-d. Right ear: endoscopic view of epitympanum with 30° angle, 2.7 mm diameter optical system. **a** Rough zone corresponding to cells; **b** main trunk of nerve of Jacobson; **c** protuberance of styloid eminence, zone of implantation; **d** zone of junction with retrotympanum

cavity, the supratubal fossula [Proctor (1964), Guerrier and Andréa (1980) and Yamasoba (1990)]. This has been called the "sinus epitympani" by Wigand and Trillsch (1973).

While its existence is virtually constant, it does vary in depth. Hoschino (1988) and Yamasoba (1990) describe three types of cavities according to the pneumatisation of the temporal bone. This region, where the internal wall is rough and studded with little spicules (fig. 16 a,b), and therefore of least resistance, allows forward extension of a cholesteatoma with ease.

Indeed, the view under the operating microscope of this supratubal fossula distal to the tegmen tympani at the level of the geniculate ganglion may lead one to overlook epidermal fragments capable of giving rise to a residual cholesteatoma, as evidenced by certain statistics: Wayoff (1982), Horn (1986).

Therefore, the use of 0° and 30° angles of vision at operation gives us a magnified view of this zone, and thus greater reliability of excision, at the completion of eradication of a cholesteatoma during the first operative stage (fig. 19).

Similarly, during the second surgical stage of a closed-technique tympanoplasty for cholesteatoma, it is advisable to check this anterior epitympanic region with the endoscope so as to exclude any residual pearl.

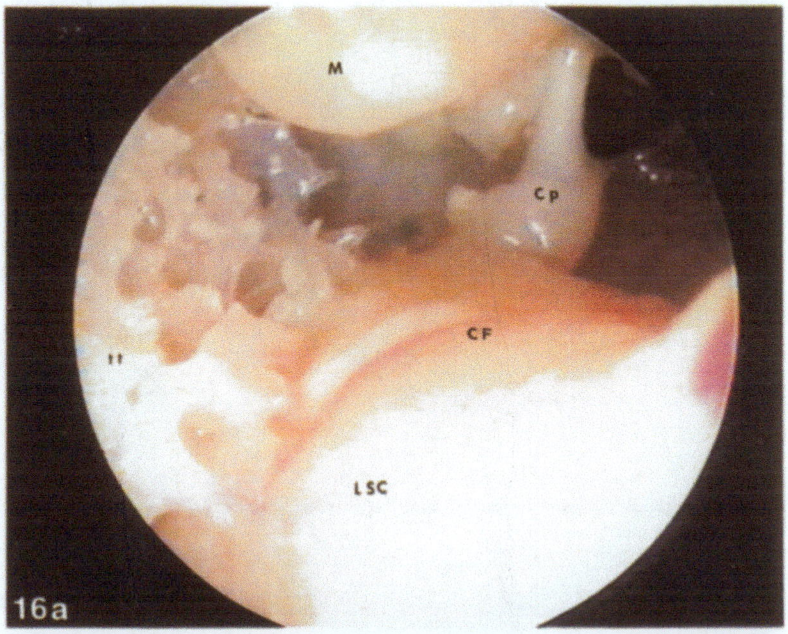

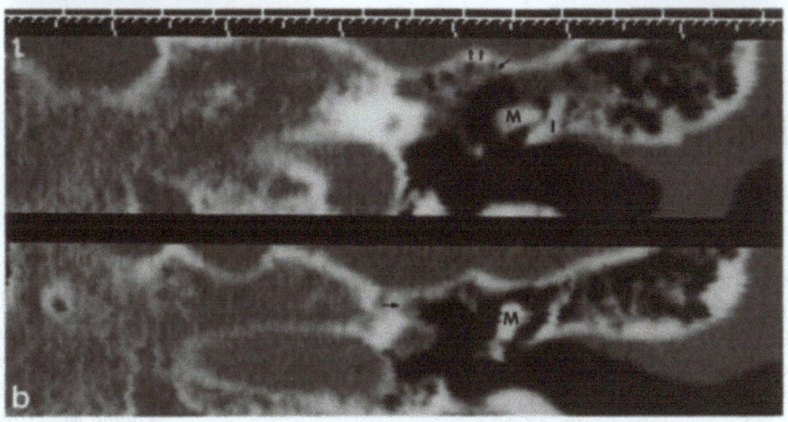

Fig. 16 a,b. View of epitympanic region (0° angle optical system) (videoprint). **a** Medial wall rough and irregular; **b** CT, frontal sections through epitympanum

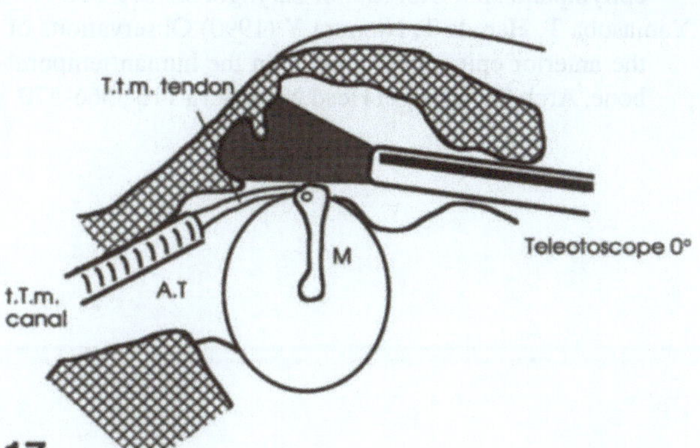

17

Fig. 17. Survey of epitympanum with 0° optical system

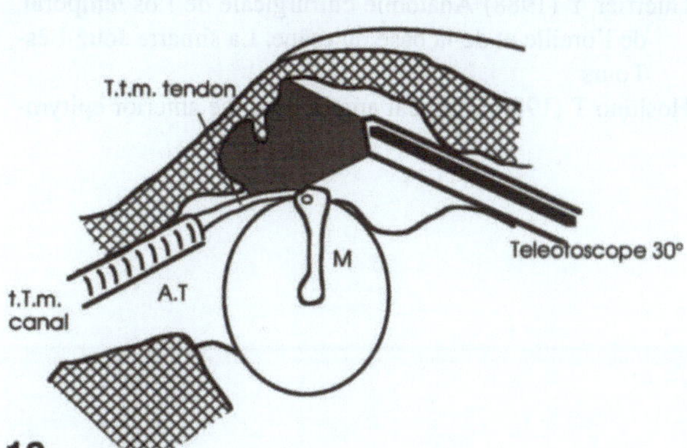

18

Fig. 18. Visual field obtained with optical system of 30°

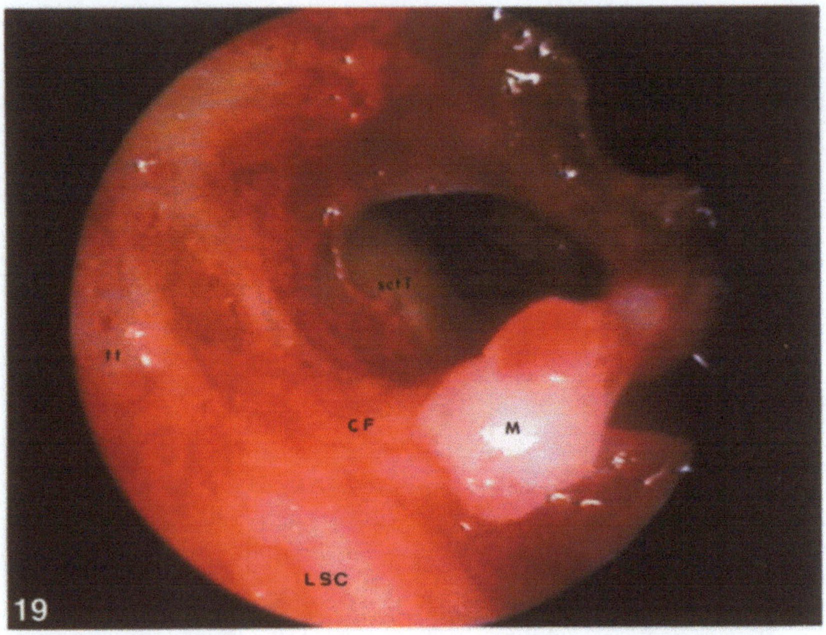

Fig. 19. Right ear: survey of anterior epitympanic region (videoprint)

References

Donalson J, Anson B, Warpeka R, Rensink M (1970) The surgical anatomy of the sinus tympani. Arch Otolaryngol, Head Neck Surg 91 : 219-227

Guerrier Y, Andrea M, Biancalana G (1976) De la paroi postérieure à la région postérieure de la caisse. Cah ORL 11 : 773-777

Guerrier Y, Andrea M (1980) Les repaires anatomiques du cholestéatome dans la caisse du tympan. Ann Otol Laryngol (Paris) 97 : 15-28

Guerrier Y (1988) Anatomie chirurgicale de l'os temporal, de l'oreille et de la base du crâne. La simarre Joué-Lès-Tours

Hoshino T (1988) Surgical anatomy of the anterior epitympanic space. Arch Otolaryngol Head Neck Surg 114 : 1143-1145

Proctor B (1964) The development of the middle ear spaces and their surgical significance. J Laryngol Otol 78 : 631-648

Proctor B (1985) The hypotympanum. Rev Laryngol Otol Rhinol (Bord) 106 : 111-116

Saito R, Igarashi M, Alford B, Guildord B (1971) Anatomical measurement of the sinus tympani. Arch Otolaryngol Head Neck Surg 94 : 418-425

Wigand M, Trillsch K (1973) Surgical anatomy of the sinus epitympani. Ann Otol Rhinol Laryngol 82 :379-383

Yamasoba T, Harada T, Nomura Y (1990) Observations of the anterior epitympanic recess in the human temporal bone. Arch Otolaryngol Head Neck Surg 116 : 566-570

Otoscopic findings

Politzer (1885) was one of the first to construct an atlas using plates from drawings to show the different appearances of the tympanic membrane. Molinie (1918) suggested stereoscopic photography of the tympanum. Later, photography using the operating microscope provided the only teaching material for many years. This was initiated by House (1959) and Myers (1961). In fact, this procedure was reserved mainly for views taken during surgical operations, and only more rarely during otoscopic examinations. Then came the advent of endoscopic photography, pioneered by Takahashi (1970) among others. This method had the advantage of bringing the objective to within less than 1 cm from the tympanic membrane.

Others elsewhere developed this technique: Buckingham (1963), Chen (1971), Chole (1980), in France, Deguine (1982) and Martin (1989). The use of flash-incorporated light sources makes available records of very high photographic quality. At present, the use of the endoscope is progressively supplanting traditional examination with speculum and forehead mirror. Only the optical system gives a wide angle of vision, not only of the entire tympanic membrane but also of the walls of the external acoustic meatus.

Three components are essential for the conduct of this examination:

– an optical sytem of 4 mm diameter, 0° angle and 60 or 100 mm in length (Storz) (fig. 20). This optical system is suitable for every external acoustic meatus except when there is malformation (stenosis). In the very small child, a 2.7 mm system with 0° angle of vision may be required

– a cold-light source with a power of 150 watts with its light cable

– a demisting fluid

Positioning the patient

Preferably, the patient is examined in the chair (fig. 21). In quite small children, otoscopy may be performed in the same way, the child being held by a third person, or else in dorsal decubitus.

Otoendoscopy

Technique

Advance of the distal lens system is achieved under visual monitoring through the external acoustic meatus. If a photographic apparatus is being used, advance of the endoscope is followed in the viewfinder, provided with frosted glass. When the endoscope is coupled to a video camera, guidance of the latter is via the screen of the video monitor.

Making photographic or videoscopic records provides a data bank which makes it easy to compare the findings of successive examinations (important in the follow-up of retraction pockets).

Decontamination of equiment

This is desirable because of the risk of transmission of hepatitis B or the HIV virus. The lens system is immersed in a 2% solution of glutamaldehyde (Sekusept®) for a period of 20 minutes, followed by rinsing in sterile water.

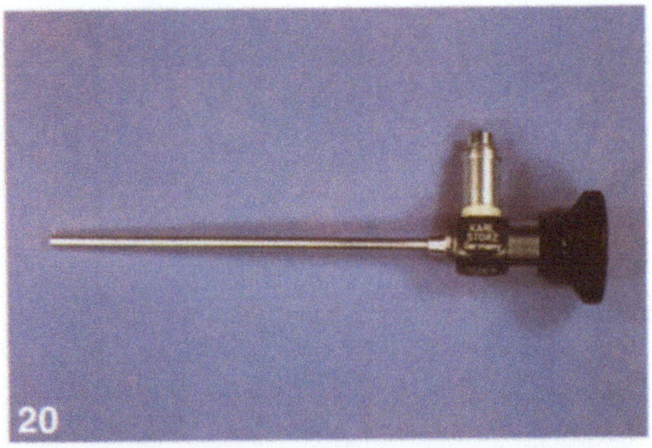

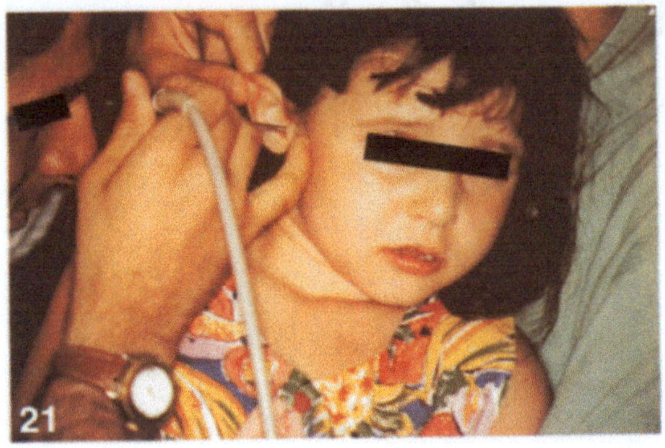

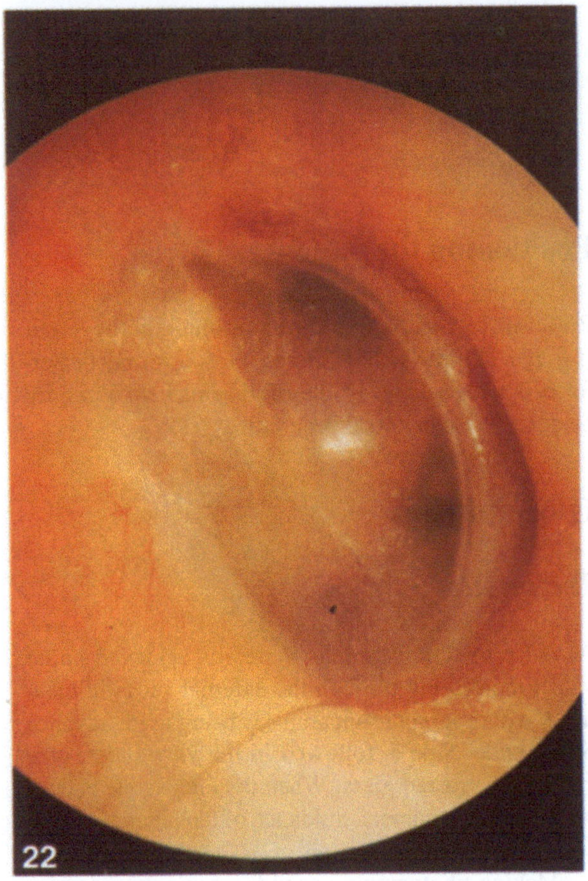

Fig. 20. Otonasopharyngoscope, 0° angle, 4 mm diameter, 100 mm long (Storz). This system allows examination of both the tympanum and the pharyngeal tubal orifice

Fig. 21. Otoscopic examination is conducted with the patient seated, as also with children

Fig. 22. Right ear: normal tympanum (objective 0° angle, 4 mm diameter)

Otoendoscopic findings

Normal eardrum

Grey in color and slightly transparent, this presents with surface irregularities (prominence of the handle of the malleus and of the lateral apophysis) (fig. 22).

Abnormal eardrum

Perforations

These constitute a solution of continuity creating a communication between the external and middle ear

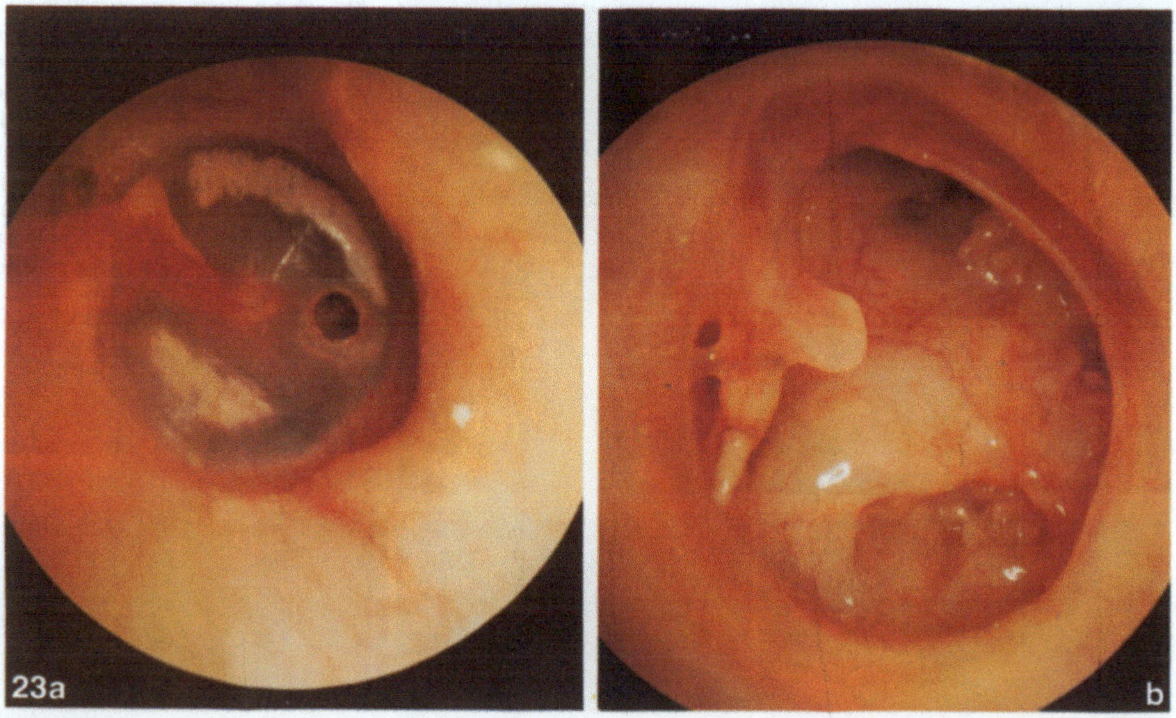

Fig. 23 a, b. Right ear: tympanic perforations. **a** Nonmarginal perforation of pars tensa; **b** Subtotal marginal perforation related to handle of malleus

(fig. 23 a, b). The insertion, in an anesthetised patient, of an endoscope through the perforation provides information as to the state of the tympanic cavity.

Retraction pockets

This is an otoscopic entity characterised by the fact that part of the tympanic membrane is no longer in the reference anatomic plane, but situated medial to this, towards the cavity of the middle ear (fig. 24 a-e).

There are three essential features to be studied concerning these pouches:

– their site, marginal or otherwise.

Though their topography varies, they are most often seen either at the posterior part of the pars tensa, where they may create a subligamentous pouch directed towards the posterior sulcus, or in the epitympanic region. In the first case there is sometimes a subtotal invagination of the whole of the pars tensa against the medial wall of the tympanic cavity.

– The quality of the covering epidermis, whether dyskeratotic or not

– the adhesion of this pocket in relation to the ossicles and the bony rim.

This is best assessed by the use of a pneumatic endoscope.

Otoscopic examination using 0° and 30° objectives provides a more precise assessment of the boundaries of the pocket than does examination with the operating microscope.

With the aim of clarification, Charachon (1988) has suggested a classification in terms of the mobility or fixity of the pouch, its site and boundaries, so as to label it as capable or not of being monitored. Nowadays, an endoscopic criterion would need to be added to this classification, depending on whether the base of the pocket can be seen with an optical system of 0°, 30° or 70°.

In our experience, endoscopic examination currently affords the best possiblility of assessing the quality of the invaginated epidermis. The keeping of photographic records ensures more precise surveillance in so-called marginal pockets or where the risks of epidermal damage are increased. According to Bremond and Magnan (1990), a retraction pocket is dangerous when it is marginal, dyskeratotic and adherent to the subjacent bony plane, since its future development cannot be monitored. In such a case, operation is indicated.

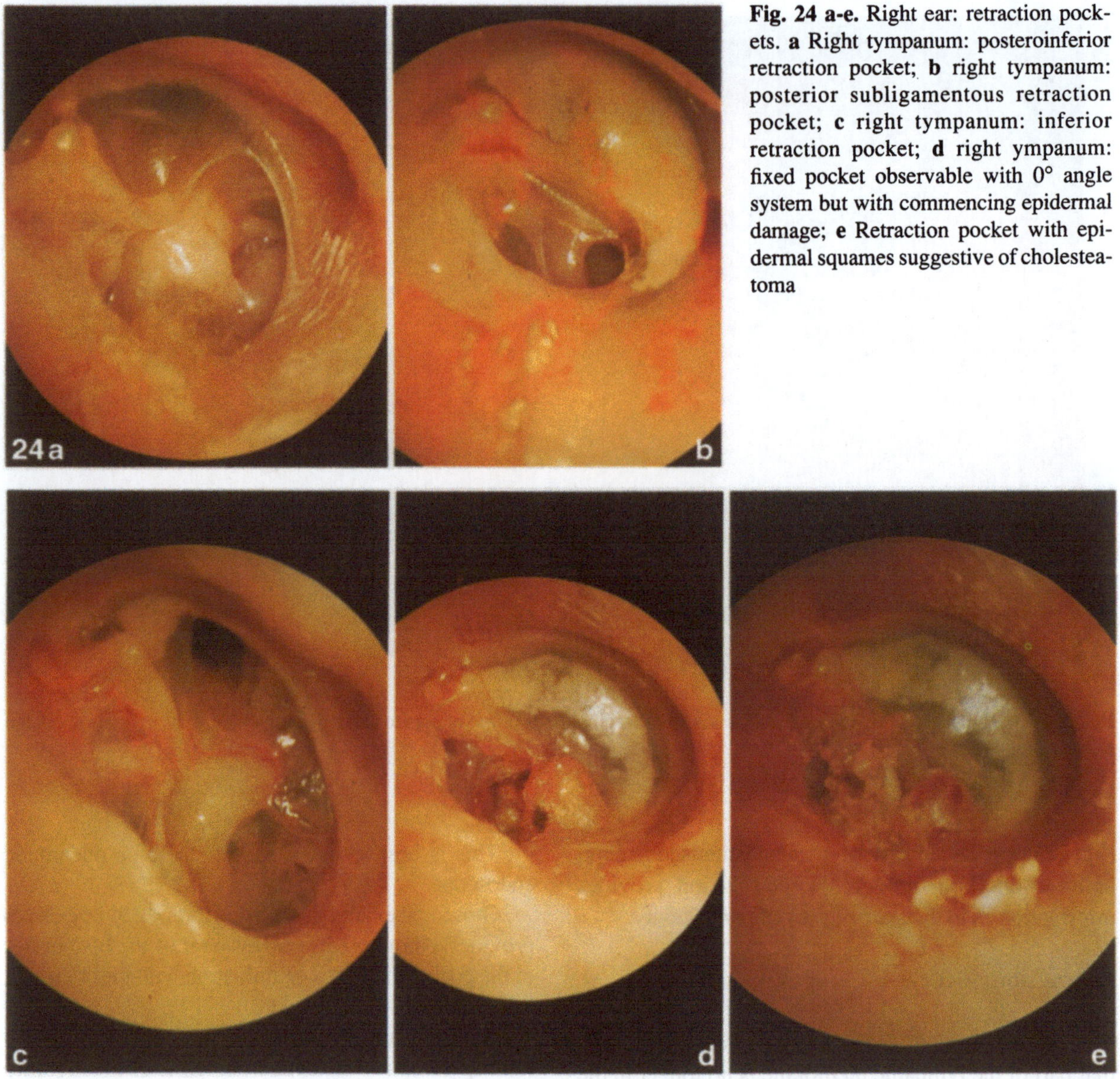

Fig. 24 a-e. Right ear: retraction pockets. **a** Right tympanum: posteroinferior retraction pocket; **b** right tympanum: posterior subligamentous retraction pocket; **c** right tympanum: inferior retraction pocket; **d** right ympanum: fixed pocket observable with 0° angle system but with commencing epidermal damage; **e** Retraction pocket with epidermal squames suggestive of cholesteatoma

Cholesteatoma

At otoscopy this appears whitish, more or less limited in extent, and with soft and friable consistency (fig. 25 a-f), Sometimes the diagnosis may be rendered more difficult by the presence of otorrhea or a sentinel polyp. Otoscopic examination must then include:

– examination using an optical stem 4 mm in diameter and 100 mm in length to visualise the entirety of the external acoustic meatus and the tympanic membrane. Some attical cholesteatomas with a normal tympanum may pass unnoticed during speculum examination

– examination with the operating microscope fitted with a focal length of 200 or 250 mm to clean out and then aspirate the accumulated squames and encrustations in the meatus or tympanic cavity.

Endoscopic anatomy of the pharyngeal orifice of the auditory tube

With the rigid optical system 4 mm in diameter and 100 mm in length used for examination of the tympanum, the pharyngeal orifice of the auditory tube can be investigated via the nasal fossa. Rotation imparted to the endoscope allows inclusion of the following anatomic parameters. When centered on the vomerine

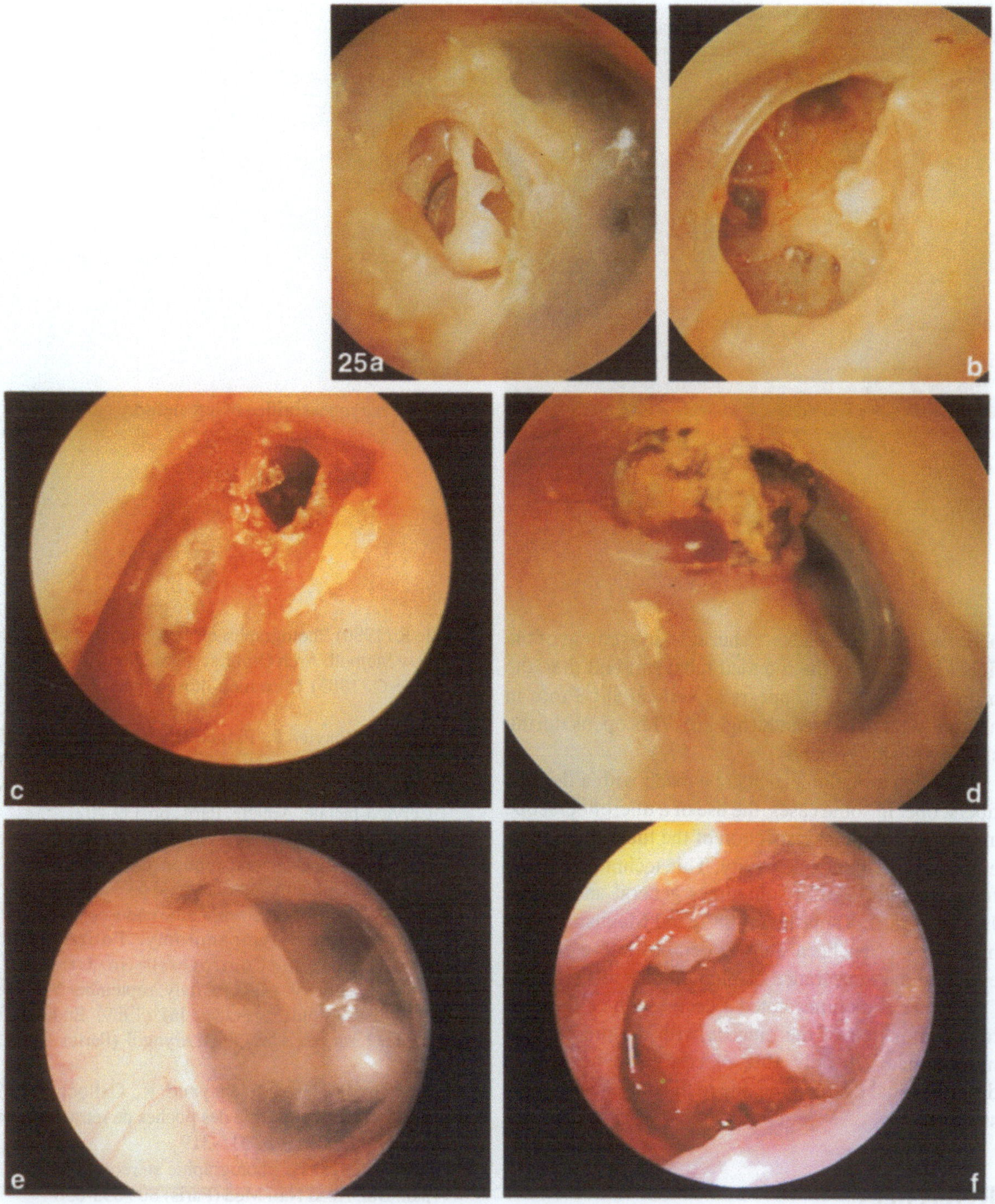

Fig. 25 a-f. Cholesteatomas. **a** Right ear: marginal perforation with epidermal cyst on superstructure of stapes; **b** left ear: subtotal marginal perforation with presence of cholesteatoma at extremity of handle of malleus; **c** left ear: perforation of pars flaccida in a child; **d** right ear: posterior attical perforation. The tympanic membrane is elevated by the cholesteatoma; **e** right ear: iatrogenic cholesteatoma after placement of transtympanic aerator (videoprint); **f** residual pearls embedded in protympanum, not visible with the operating microscope (videoprint)

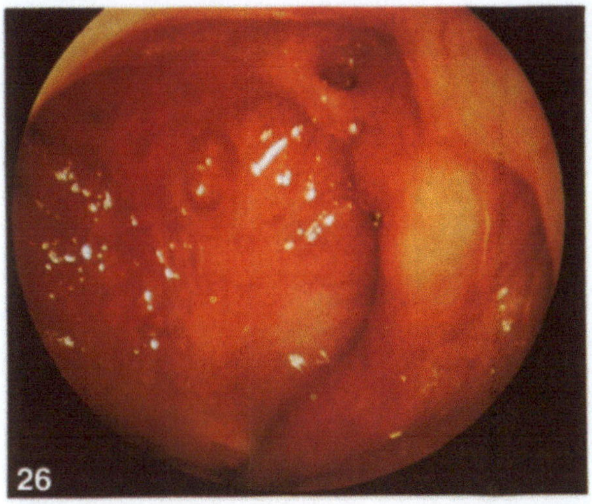

Fig. 26. Pharyngeal orifice of left auditory tube

plate, with the choanae on either side, movement of the fiberscope locates the rounded tubal rim and then the orifice, which at rest appears as vertical slit 8 mm in height by 1 mm in breadth (fig. 26). This opens during swallowing movements

This examination can also be made with a flexible fiberscope. In some cases, the use of a microfiberscope allows endoluminal inspection of the tube as far as its entry into the tympanic cavity. This technique is performed under local or sometimes general anesthesia. Jansen (1986), Yamashita (1989) and Magnan (1990) have very often been able to demonstrate a normal endoluminal appearance of the auditory tube. Jansen (1986) has sometimes noted a decrease in caliber due to inflammation of the mucosa with the presence of much mucus. In only 10% of cases was he able to describe tubal dysfunction due to the presence of bony stenosis.

References

Bremond G, Magnan J, Chays A, Florence A, Gignac D, Lebreuil G (1990) Les poches de rétraction, entité pathologique ? Ann Otol Laryngol (Paris) 107 : 386-392

Buckingham R (1963) Endoscopic otophotography. Laryngoscope 73 : 71-84

Charachon R (1988) Classification des poches de rétraction. Rev Laryngol Otol Rhinol (Bord) 109 : 205-207

Chen B, Fry T, Fischer N (1979) Otoscopy and photography. Ann Otol Rhinol Laryngol 88 : 771-773

Chole R (1980) Photography of the tympanic membrane. A new Method. Arch Otol Laryngol 106 : 230-231

Deguine C (1983) L'examen otoscopique. NPN Médecine 52 : 2

Freche Ch, Rouvier P, Piquet JJ, Thomassin JM (1989) Endoscopie diagnostique et thérapeutique en ORL. Rapport à la Société Française d'ORL de Pathologie Cervico-faciale. Arnette, Paris, pp 339-402

House W, House H, Urban J (1959) Operating microscope observation viewer and motion picture camera. Trans Am Acad Ophtalmol Otolaryngol 63 : 228-229

Jansen C (1986) New eustachia tube endoscope without and with posterior tympanotomy. Politzer Society Conference on Controversis in Otology and Otoneurosurgery, Alghero, Italy, september 1-6, 1986

Martin Ch, Mayaud R, Prades JM (1989) Endoscopie et cophochirurgie. Ann Otol Laryngol (Paris) 106 : 523-524

Martin Ch, Prades JM, Mayaud R, Calloch F (1993) Endoscopie et chirurgie des poches de rétraction tympaniques. J Fr ORL 42 : 315-319

Molinie M (1918) La photographie stéréoscopique du tympan. Bull Acad Natl Med (Paris) 80 : 655-656

Myers D (1960) Photography during otologic microsurgery. Med Radiogr Photogr 36 : 45-62

Politzer A (1885) Die Beleuchtungsbilder des Trommelfells im gesunden und kranken Zusttarde. Wilhem Braumuller, Wien

Takahashi F (1966) Communication personnelle. Acta Otorhinol Laryngola Belg 29 : 270-271

Thomassin JM, Korchia D (1992) Examen clinique de l'oreille. In : Encyclop Med Chir ORL, 20025A10 Paris, 5 p

Instrumentation

Surgery under endoscopic guidance and video monitoring is a new technique in the field of otology. It has necessitated the development of teleotoscopes of appropriate diameter and length, while conforming to the requirements of the optical components involved in their manufacture. As regards their diameter for use via the EAM, our anatomic studies have shown that the distance between the handle of the malleus and the bony margin of the acoustic meatus always exceeds 3 mm (fig. 27). Hence, we chose a diameter of 2.7 mm.

The insertion of these optical systems by a posterior route to survey the antro-attical passage or the tympanic cavity via the window of a posterior tympanotomy (breadth 3 to 4 mm depending on the burring) also allows the use of a 2.7 mm system.

As to length, we have deliberately chosen short systems of 50 to 60 mm in length, thus avoiding the problem that, when connected to a micro-camera, they exert an excessive leverage on the operator's left hand. For this reason, we advise against the use of endoscopes devised for nasal sinus surgery. They are too long and are therefore dangerous.

Endoscopes

For tympanic endoscopy

We recommend two optical systems:

– a direct vision teleotoscope, 4 mm in diameter and 10 cm in length (Storz), without a protective sheath, called the otonasopharyngoscope. It allows examination of both the tympanic membrane and the pharyngeal orifice of the auditory tube by the nasal route.

– an otoendoscope of 0° angle, 2.7 mm diameter and 6 cm length, valuable for use in children or in cases of a narrow EAM.

For otovideoendoscopic surgery of the cavities of the middle ear

The surgeon must have at his disposal three optical systems whose technical characteristics give a full-screen image on the video monitor. These are 2.7 mm diameter optical systems with angles of 0°, 30° and 70° (Storz) (fig. 28 a-d). The 70° teleotoscope can explore the entirety of the cavities of the retrotympanum (sinus tympani) whatever their depths.

The endoscopes are arranged on the instrument table, in a support to protect them from shocks (fig. 29). A demisting fluid is essential. The surgeon must take care to clean the lenses every time before use.

Cold-light source

A cold-light source, fitted with two outlets of 250 watts power, is necessary with optical systems of 2.7 mm diameter.

Cold-light cable

A Y-shaped cable, with two outlets and one inlet, ensures light transmission between the generator and the endoscope.

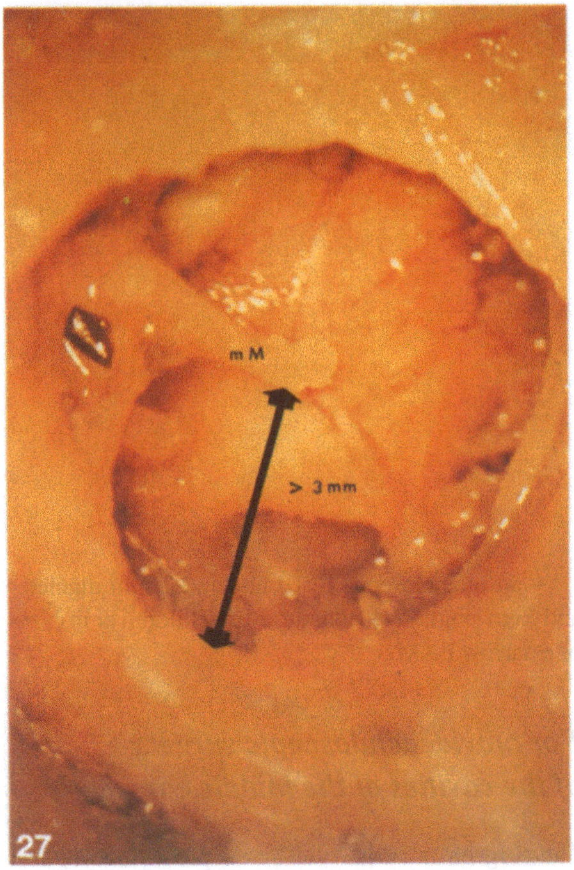

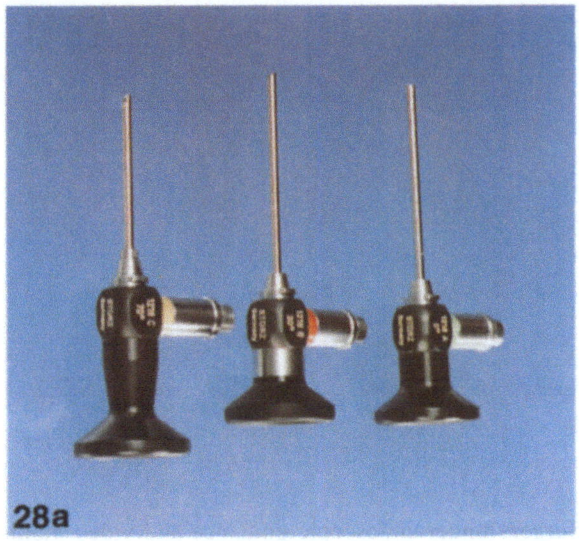

Fig. 27. Right ear: tympanic cavity (anatomic specimen)

Fig. 28 a-d. Otoendoscopes for video-monitored surgery. **a** Optical systems; **b** optical system with 0° angle; **c** optical system with 30° angle, suitable for easily accessed tympanic sinuses; **d** optical system with 70° angle, essential for difficultly accessed tympanic sinuses

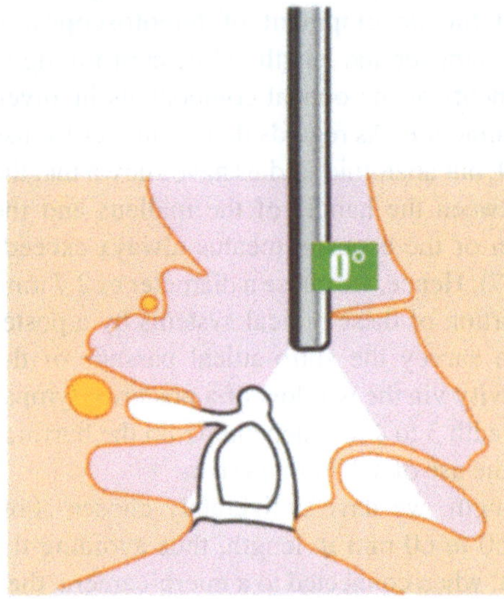

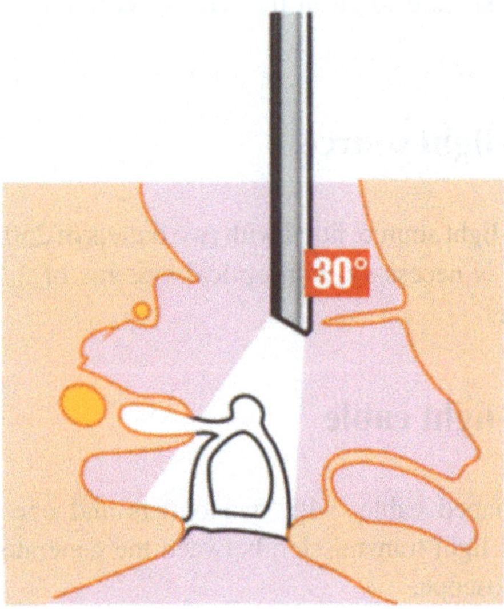

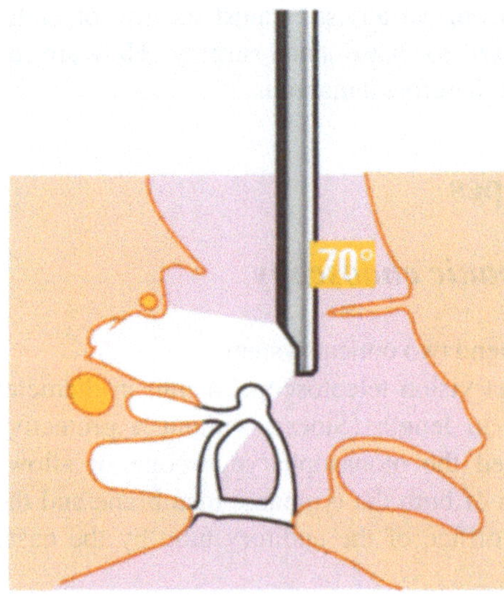

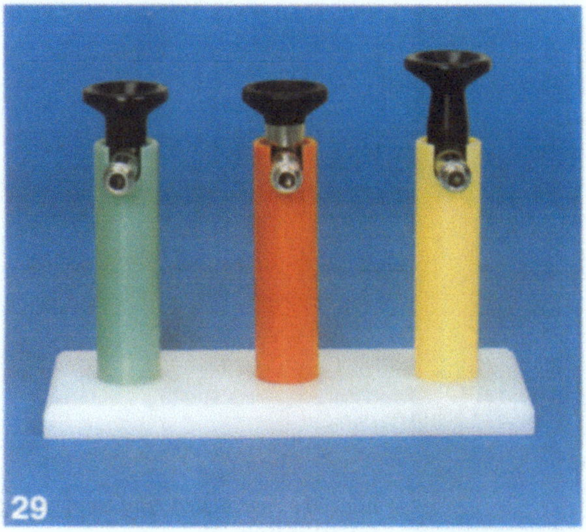

Fig. 29. Otoendoscopes in their support. Each color indicates the angulation of the optical systems

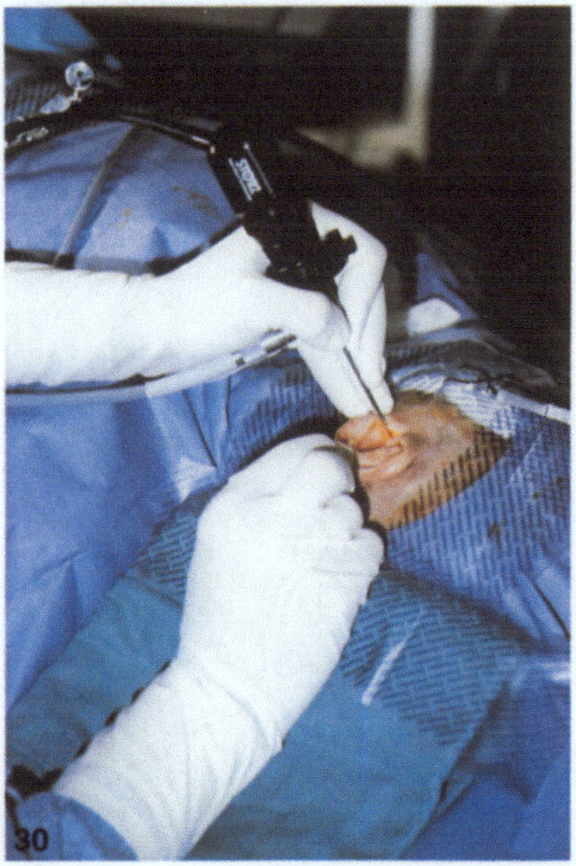

Fig. 30. The endoscope is connected to a micro-camera

Micro-camera

This must possess certain ergonomic features: it must be light, very sensitive, and provided with a zoom lens which gives an enlarged image on the monitor (fig. 30). All these features are essential if it is to be easy and suitable for use. It may be water-tight but this is not essential. However,if this is not the case, it should be precautionarily wrapped in a sterile covering.

Support of the optical system

In certain tympanoplasties for cholesteatoma where the handle of the malleus is no longer present, it is possible to fix the optical system coupled to the camera by means of an articulated arm (fig. 31) at the tympanic cavity. The surgery of the posterior region of the tympanic cavity then becomes easier, since the surgeon has both hands available for use.

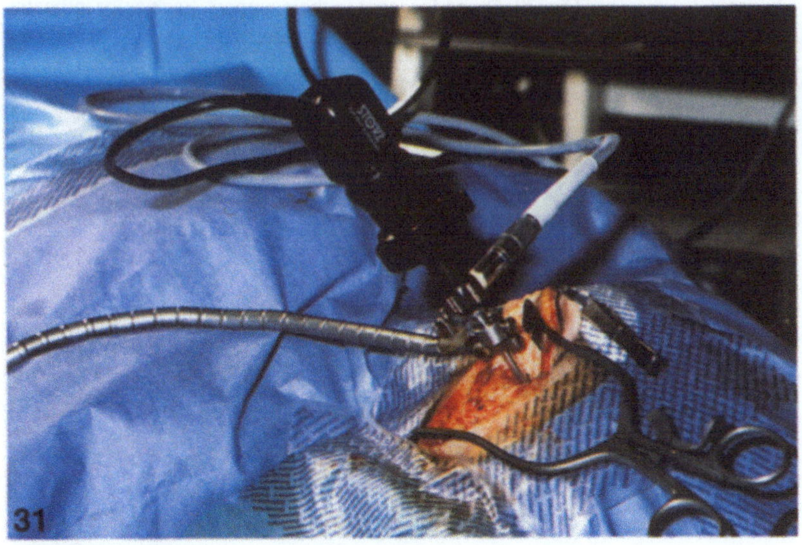

31

Fig. 31. Articulated arm supporting optical system

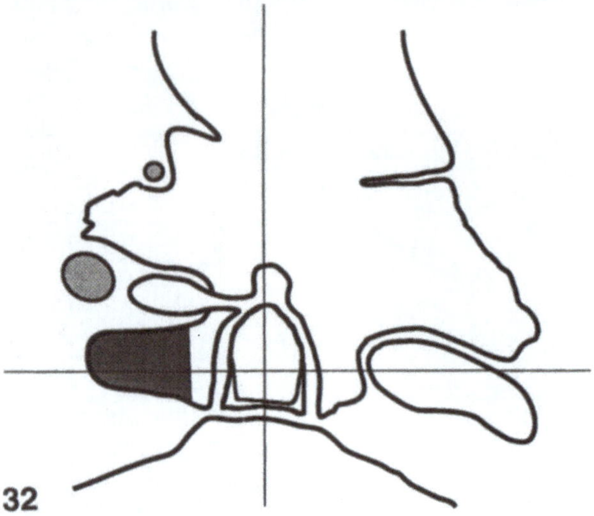

32

Fig. 32. Sagittal section through tympanic cavity

Decontamination and sterilisation of equipment

The micro-camera is immersed in a decontaminating agent such as 0.5% ampholysine plus for 15 minutes. It is then rinsed, immersed in the same fluid, and rinsed again in sterile water. It may be safely stored in a box containing pastilles of formaldehyde. It is recommended that the endoscopes be soaked in the same 0.5% solution of ampholysine plus. Then, after rinsing and washing with sterile water, they are finally sterilised in an autoclave at 2 kg pressure at a temperature of 138° for 15 minutes.

Micro-instruments

Specific instrumentation is essential for surgery of the retrotympanum. It is a fact that excision of diseased tissue from the posterior tympanic region is difficult. The different fossulae it contains have an axis perpendicular to that of the external acoustic meatus. They are also in a recessed situation relative to the bony margin of the tympanic setting (fig. 32).

The use of an optical system directed obliquely at 70° requires the use of micro-instruments angled at 90° for access to this region.

The instrument set (Storz) includes (fig. 33 a-c):

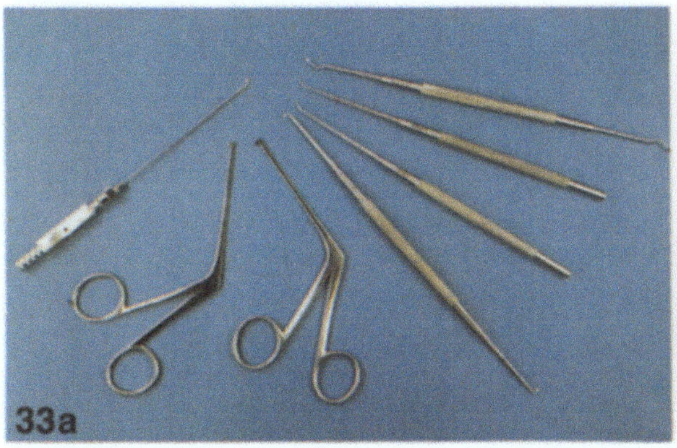

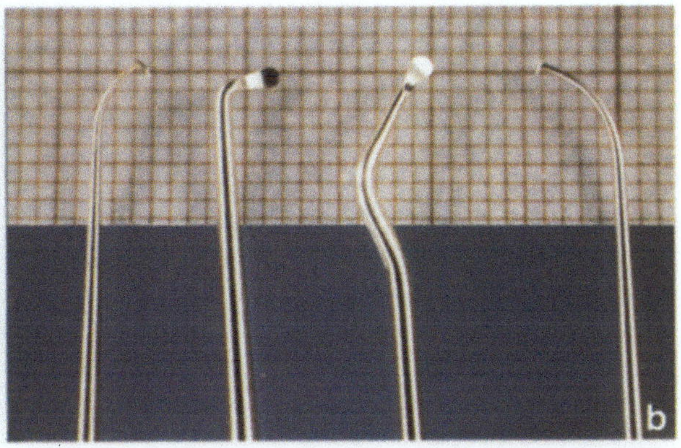

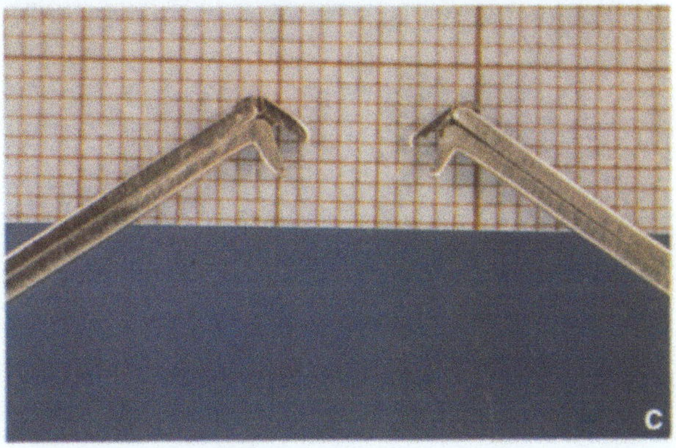

Fig. 33a-c. Equipment. **a** Set of instruments; **b** micro-hook, dissector and rugine; **c** micro-forceps with hollow and grooved jaws, angled at 90°

– a double micro-dissector, one end of which is bent to the right and the other to the left

– a curved micro-hook, bent at 90°

– a micro-rugine

– a support for the micro-suckers

– micro-suckers of 0.6, 0.8 and 1 mm diameter

– micro-forceps bent at 90° with hollow (punch) and grooved jaws

Endoscopic guided surgery with video monitoring

Anesthesia

General anesthesia – technique

(Conciatori J MD, Rud C MD, Vilcoq P MD)

Microsurgery of the middle ear requires a bloodless operative field. Any bleeding that may occur during such surgery, performed with microscopes or endoscopes, can hinder and endanger eradication of the disease process. The techniques for reduction of hemorrhage (controlled arterial hypotension) must ensure a bloodless operative field, while remaining rapidly reversible.

Preoperative period

Premedication alleviates stress factors and prepares the patient for operation., Therefore one hour before beginning the operation benzodiazepam (xanax) is given together with a conversion enzyme inhibitor (CEI)(lopril 25 mg) orally for certain patients.

Operative period

Induction is made using pentothal (0.8 mg/kg), norcuron (0.1 mg/kg) and fentanyl) (0,2 mg/kg) combined with antibiotic cover (augmentin)(1 g IV slowly).

Intubation is performed with a preformed tube. Maintenance of general anesthesia is obtained with a combination of fentanyl and forene. Forene is the most commonly used hypotensive agent. Its vasodilator action exists in concentrations of 0.5 to 5%. It is reversible with moderate tachycardia, and without affecting the cardiac output. This anesthetic is potentiated by CEIs, which allows the dosage to be considerably reduced. Severe arterial hypotension requires infusion with Ringer lactate solution and vasopressors (ephedrine).

In 25% of cases, where is resistance even to high concentrations of forene, recourse to other medications is advised:

– beta-blockers, particularly labetolol (trandate) in a total (fractionated) dose of 0.3 mg/kg;

– esmolol (breviblocR=), which has a very rapid but also transient action, as a bolus of 200-500 gamma/kg;

– an alpha-blocker, urapidil (eupressyl) in a dose of 25 mg in 25 seconds.

Postural drainage is promoted by tilting the head and chest upward by 15 to 20° to the horizontal.

Monitoring

This is very important and is effected by electrocardiographic monitoring, measurement of arterial pressure and oscillometry, avoiding sudden variations in systolic pressure, which should lie between 70 and 90 mm Hg (average 60 mm Hg), and by pulse oximetry (SaO_2 98%).

Measurement of CO_2 levels (capnometry) allows adjustment of the ventilation (FiO_2 0.5) so as to prevent any hypercapnia, a cause of arterial hypertension.

Recovery

Thanks to the reduced use of morphinic agents, recovery is rapid and satisfactory and cough is avoided dur-

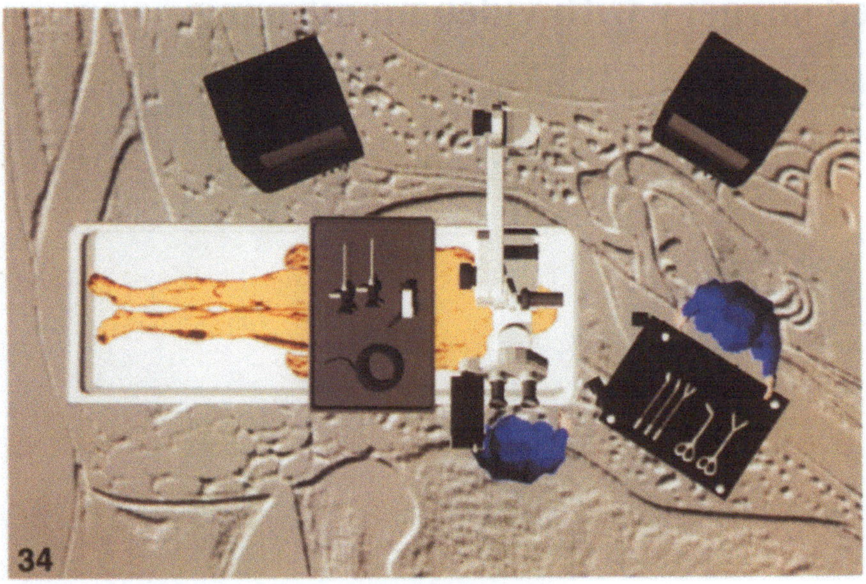

Fig. 34. Arrangement of operating room

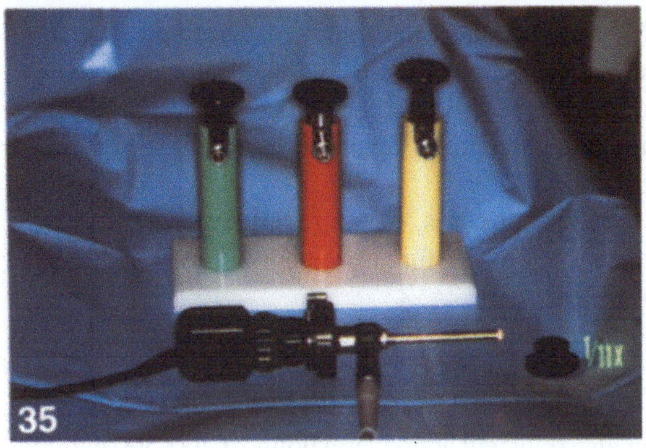

Fig. 35. Endoscopes of 0°, 30° and 70° angles in their support

ing extubation. The arterial pressure rapidly returns to normal, so that it is wise to restrict the duration of hypotension to that period when it is useful to the surgeon.

Local anesthesia

Local anesthesia by infiltration is the method most commonly employed. The injection of 2 to 3 ml of lidocaine (2%) with adrenalin into the posterior part of the EAM at the boundary of the pilo-sebaceous zone, supplemented by injection of the anterior part of the meatus, allows exploration of the tympanic cavity via the channel during the second operative stage. At the same time, the retroauricular region is infiltrated with 2% lidocaine at two or three sites.

This technique is employed for inspection of the posterior cavities under video monitoring by a minimal retroauricular skin incision (cf chapter on technique). To reduce minor operative bleeding, small pieces of gelfoam soaked in adrenalin can be used. These are applied to the hemorrhagic area for one or two minutes.

Arrangement of operating room and patient (fig. 34)

The patient is supine, in dorsal decubitus, with his head turned to the opposite side. The region of the external ear and mastoid are placed directly under the vision of the surgeon, who is seated at the head of the table on the right or left side.

The foot of the operating microscope is opposite the surgeon. The articulated arm is carried as a bridge over the head. It is always fitted with a television camera. The instrument nurse is at the head of the table, with the instrument table alongside. An instrument tray supported by a single leg is situated above the

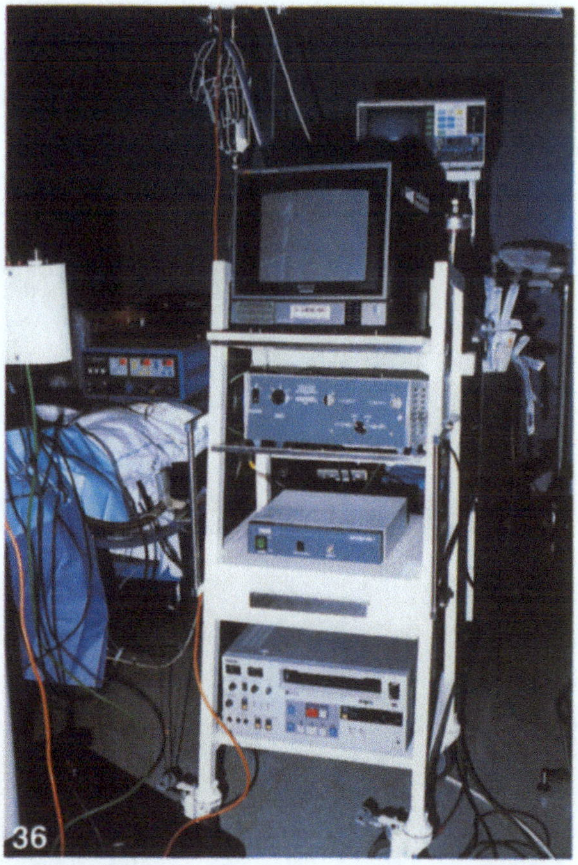

Fig. 36. Video stand housing audiovisual equipment

patient's abdomen. On it are arranged the micro-camera, the optical support with endoscopes of 0°, 30° and 70°, and the cold-light cable (fig. 35), as well as a small dish containing unwoven compresses with a demisting agent.

Finally, a stand housing the video monitor, the cold-light source, the camera-feed and the magnetoscope is installed opposite the surgeon to the left of the base of the microscope (fig. 36).

During endoscopic guided surgery, the arm of the microscope is displaced sideways and the surgeon works while watching the video monitor screen (fig. 37). An electronic control box with a simple button allows transfer from the micro-camera set-up coupled to the endoscope to the camera of the operating microscope.

The set of micro-instruments designed for surgery of the retrotympanum is arranged on the table of the instrument nurse. The operative towels are arranged all around the mastoid region in the usual manner, after an antiseptic solution has been applied around the ear, over the auricle and the meatus, except for the EAM.

A local anesthetic infiltration with a vasoconstrictor (adrenalised xylocaine: 1 ampoule of adrenaline in 40 ml of 0.5% xylocaine) is made in the periauricular region at at the EAM by the surgeon. This always precedes the skin incision.

Surgical techniques

Surgery of cholesteatoma

First operative stage of tympanoplasty by closed technique

Otoendosocopic lesional assessment

Under general anesthesia, the procedure begins with cleansing of the EAM through a speculum using the operating microscope. Then we routinely insert an endoscope with a 0° angle of vision and 4 mm in diameter to make a more precise assessment of the tym-

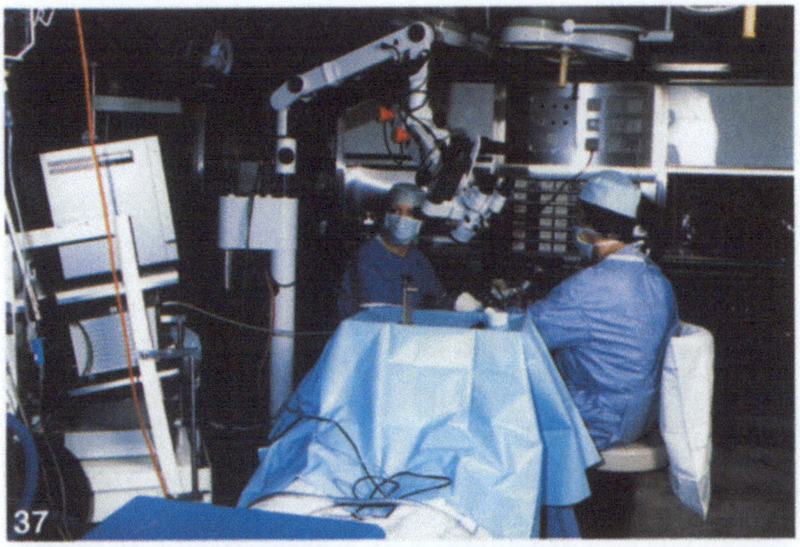

Fig. 37. During endoscopic guided surgery the operator works using a video monitor screen

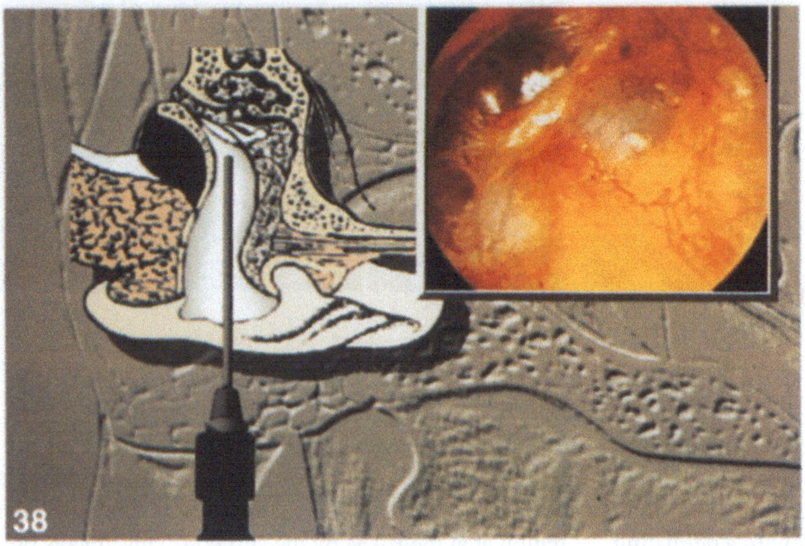

Fig. 38. Otoscopic view of tympanum, 0° angle system

panic lesions (fig. 38). If there is a major perforation of the tympanic membrane, we make use of this aperture to insert an endoscope of 0° and then, sometimes, of 30° and 70°, in order to visualise the incudo-stapedian region (figs.39 a-d, 40 a-d). Unfortunately, the presence of otorrhea or a sentinel polyp makes this examination impossible.

Peroperative otoendoscopy

The posterior approach is by far that most commonly used. Through a retroauricular skin incision and after stripping of the external ear, a mainly musculo-periosteal flap is constructed with an anterior hinge. This is then rugined to widely expose the bony mastoid

→

Fig. 39 a-d. Right ear: posterior tympanic perforation (videoprint). **a** Perforated tympanum (lens system of 30°, 2.7 mm diameter); **b, c** through the perforation the incudo-stapedial region and sinus tympani are visible; **d** the hypotympanic recess with the nerve of Jacobson.

Fig. 40 a-d. Left ear: tympanic perforation (videoprint). **a, b** Posterior perforation (optical system 70°, 2.7 mm); **c, d** region of retrotympanum (30°, 2.7 mm)

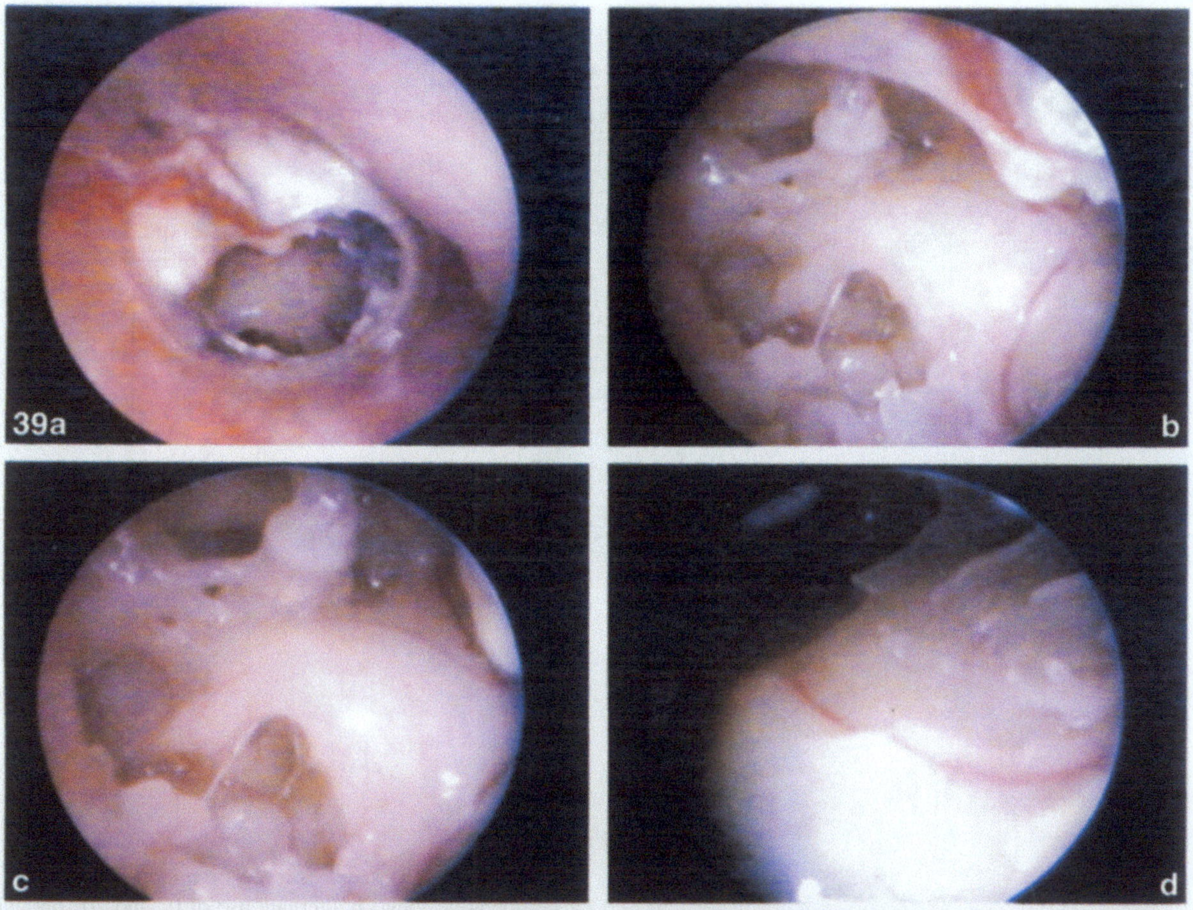
39a
b
c
d

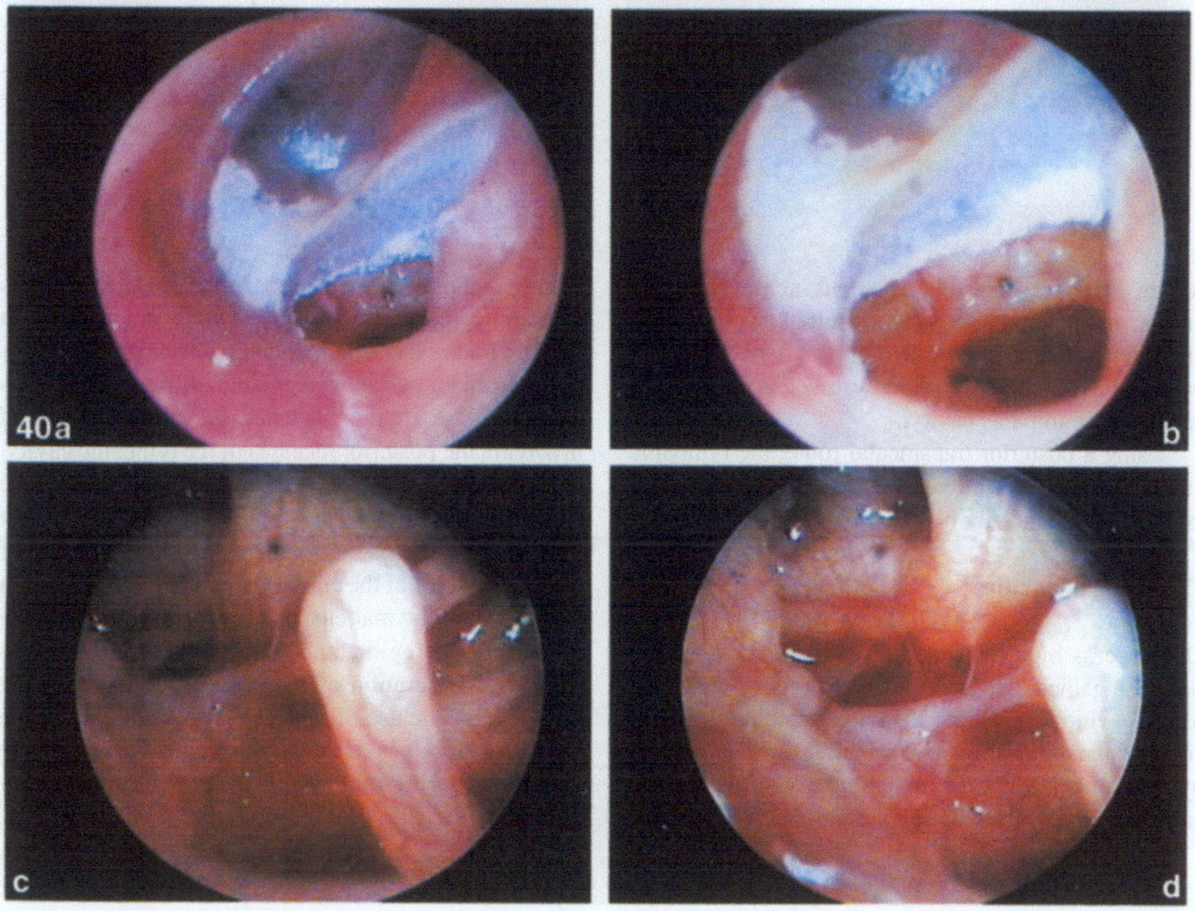
40a
b
c
d

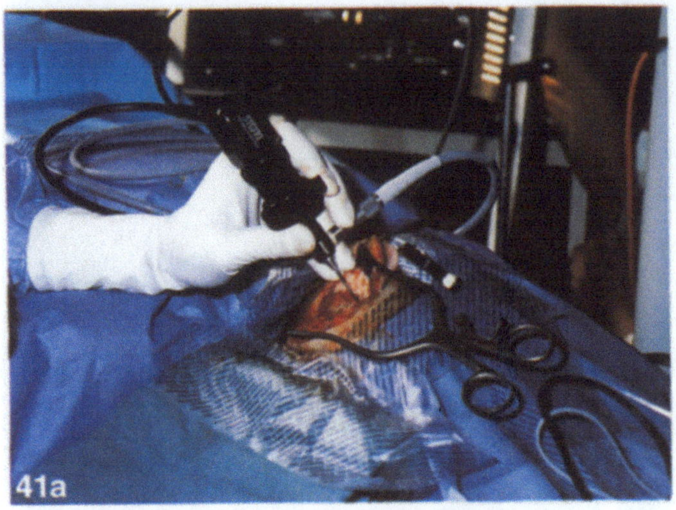

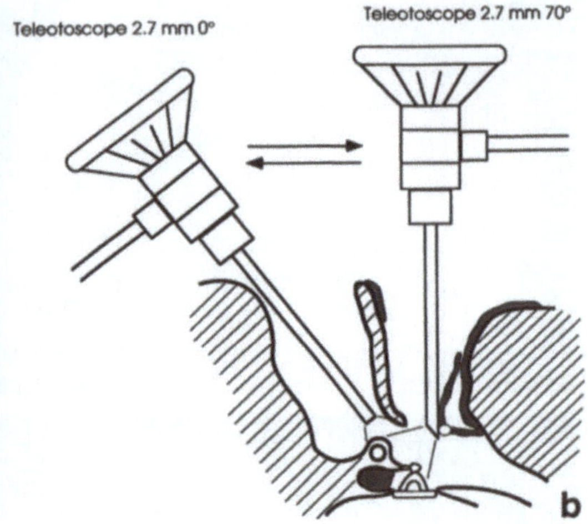

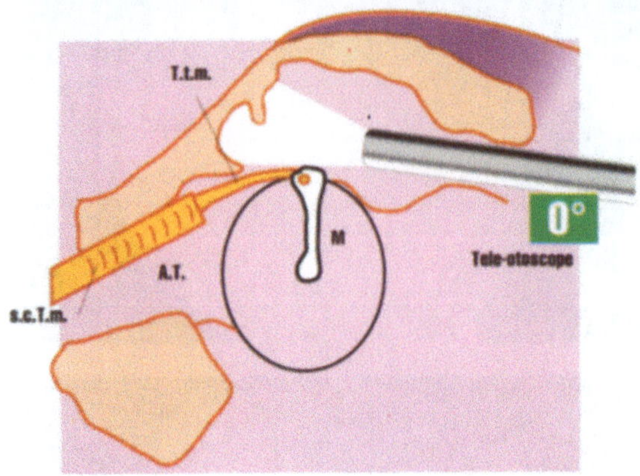

Fig. 41 a, b. Endoscopic survey of middle ear cavities. **a** Peroperative view; **b** alternate use of 0° and 70° optical systems for the middle ear cavities

Fig. 42. Diagram showing use of 0° angle endoscope in monitoring the anterior part of the epitympanum

region. The transmastoid route us achieved using cutting and diamond burrs. The result of this burring is an extensive mastoido-antro-epitympanectomy. A posterior tympanotomy window gives access to the region of the tmpanic cavity.

Using a posterior transmeatal route, the tympanic cavity is approached after stripping of a tympano-meatal flap with an inferior hinge.

Cleansing of cavities

Once access by a transmastoid and transmeatal route has been gained, the surgeon can proceed to cleansing of the cavities containing the cholesteatoma. Its excision is done according to the principles well laid down by Marquet (1989), from behind forwards, in the endeavor to eradicate the cholesteatomatous sac as a whole, without fragmentation. In the epidermosis, this monobloc dissection is not always practicable. It increases the risks of a residual cholesteatoma, developing from an overlooked epidermal fragment. This is also the case in the presence of epidermal spread involving the posterior recesses of the tympanic cavity.

Very often, the body of the incus is found to be embedded in the cholesteatoma. If this is the case, it involves its ablation during the procedure. Exposure of the anterior part of the epitympanum requires resection of the head of the malleus. this facilitates the dissection of this deep region and is also recommended to improve the aeration of the posterior cavities of the middle ear. The use of optical systems connected to a video camera does not take place until the end of the operation, during monitoring for excision of the epidermal matrix (fig. 41 a,b).

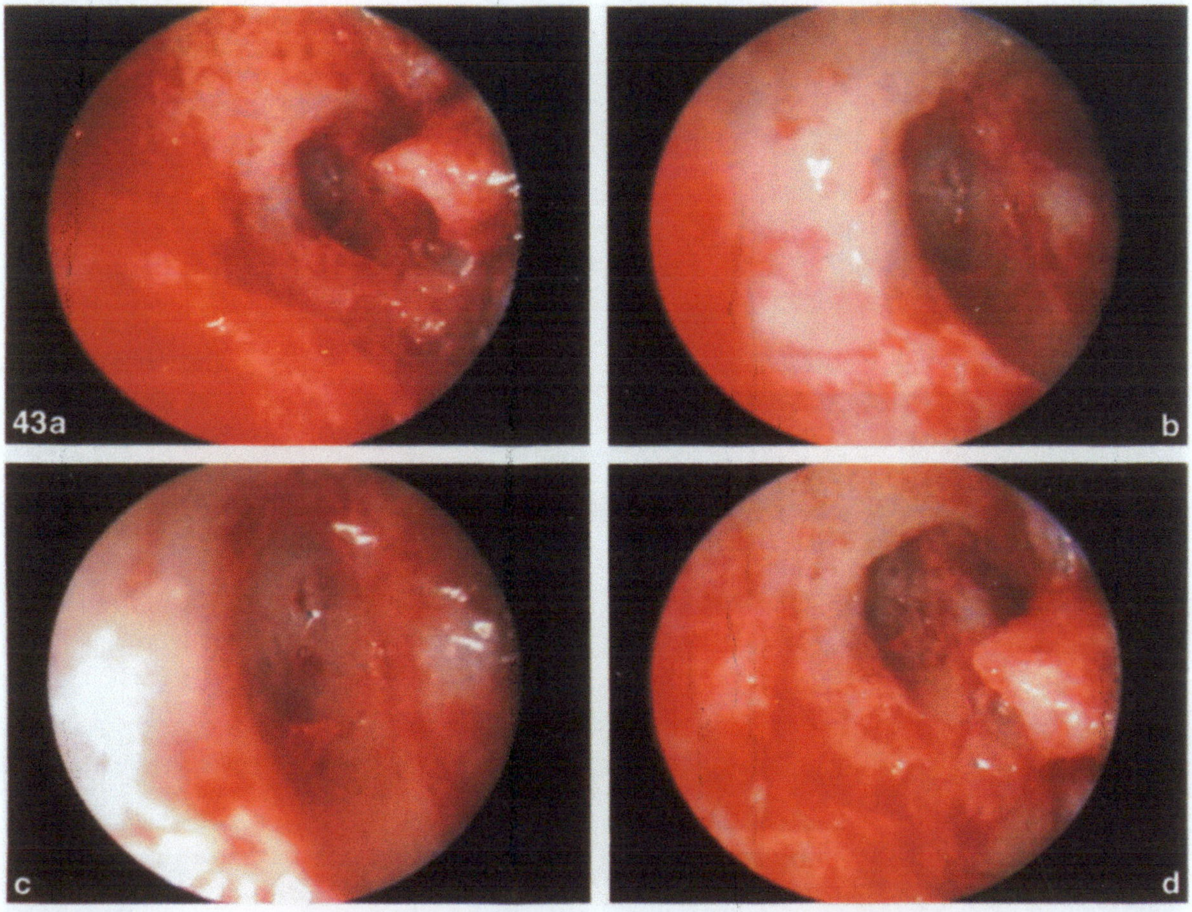

Fig. 43 a-d. Right ear: peroperative monitoring with 0° angle optical system of the anterior part of the epitympanum after excision of the cholesteatomous matrrix (videoprint). **a** Epitympanic corridor; **b-d** survey of supratubal fossula

Three zones are more particularly inspected:
– the epitympanum and supratubal fossula
– the protympanum
– the retrotympanum.

The degree of illumination and the wide angle of vision now available allow a more precise assessment in those regions, such as the retrotympanum, where access is more difficult and where visualisation with the operating microsocope may even be impossible.

Inspection of epitympanum

We begin by making an inspection of the most anterior part of the epitympanum 9 (fig. 42) using optical systems of 2.7 mm diameter and with angles of 0° and 30°. The camera fitted with an endoscope is inserted into the antro-epitympanic passage, after irrigation and *placement* of adrenalised gelfoam to reduce peroperative bleeding as much as possible.

Movement of the objective, followed on the video monitor screen, surveys all the walls of the epitympanum, especially the superior and inferior walls of the anterior attic, in the search for an epidermal microfragment which may have been overlooked at dissection under the operating microscope (figs. 43 a-d, 44 a-d). If there is the slightest doubt, a mico-instrument can be used to verify the presence or absence of epidermal tissue. If such is present, excision can be done under either endoscopic or microscopic monitoring to complete eradication.

Inspection of protympanum

A 2.7 mm, 0° angle optical system is introduced via the EAM into the tympanic cavity. It is advanced in the direction of the orifice of the auditory tube (fig. 45 a-d). Monitoring is sometimes necessary when the cholesteatoma possesses prolongations in the direction of the

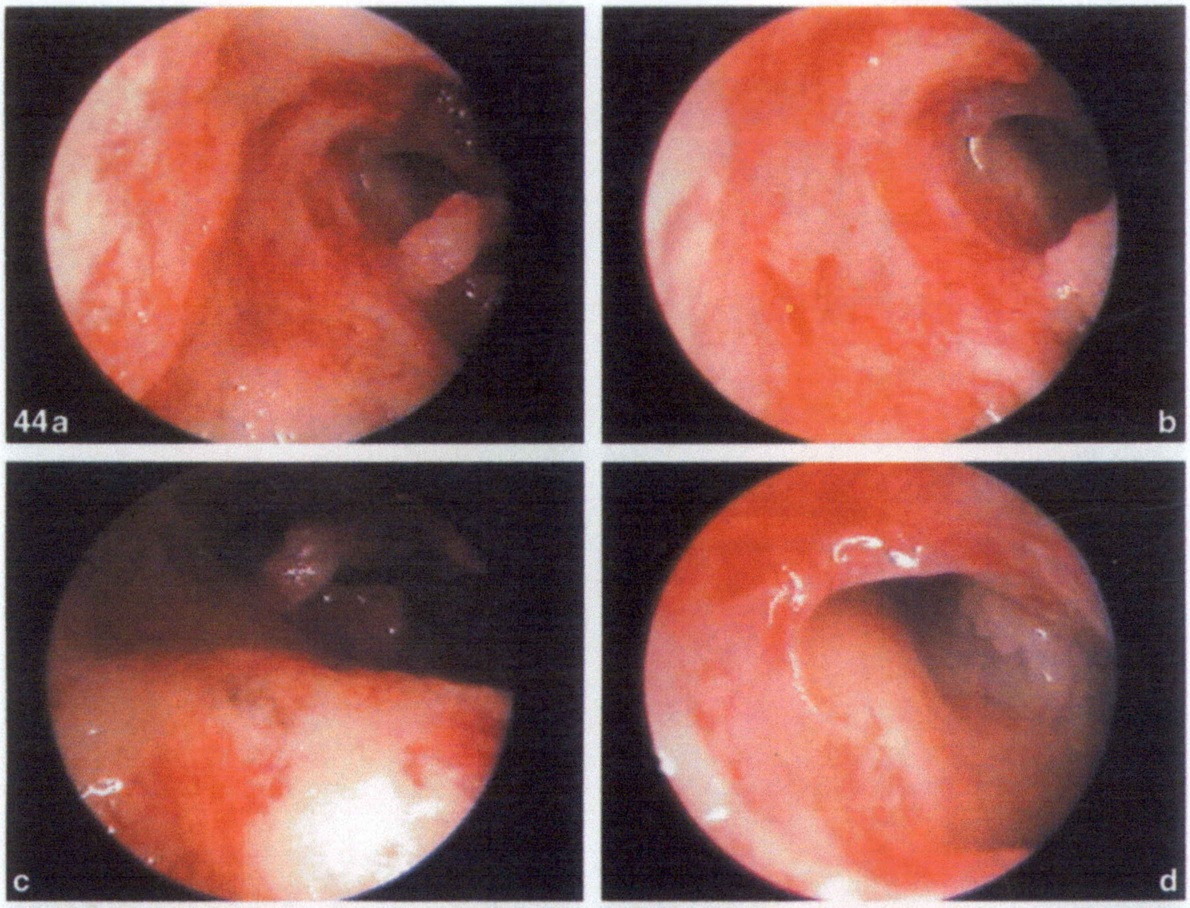
44a
b
c
d

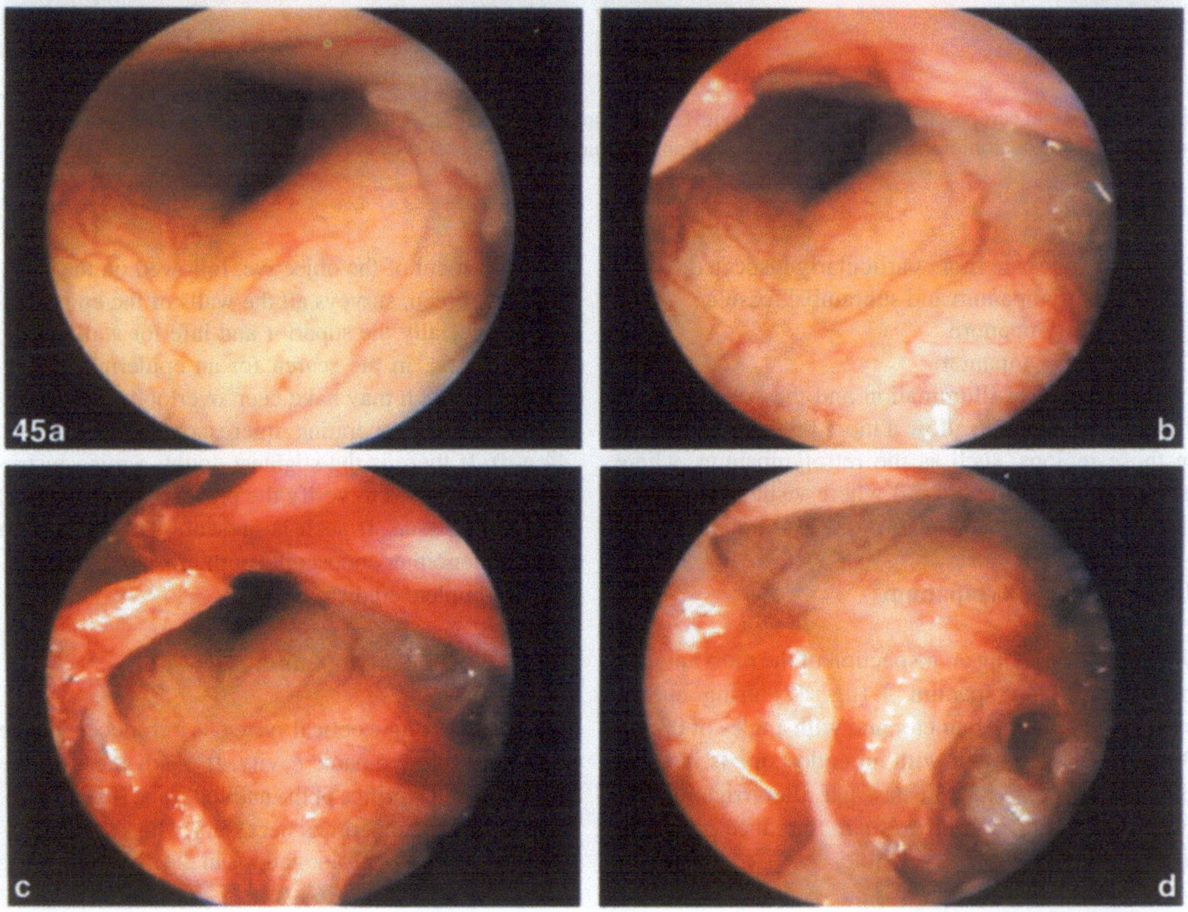
45a
b
c
d

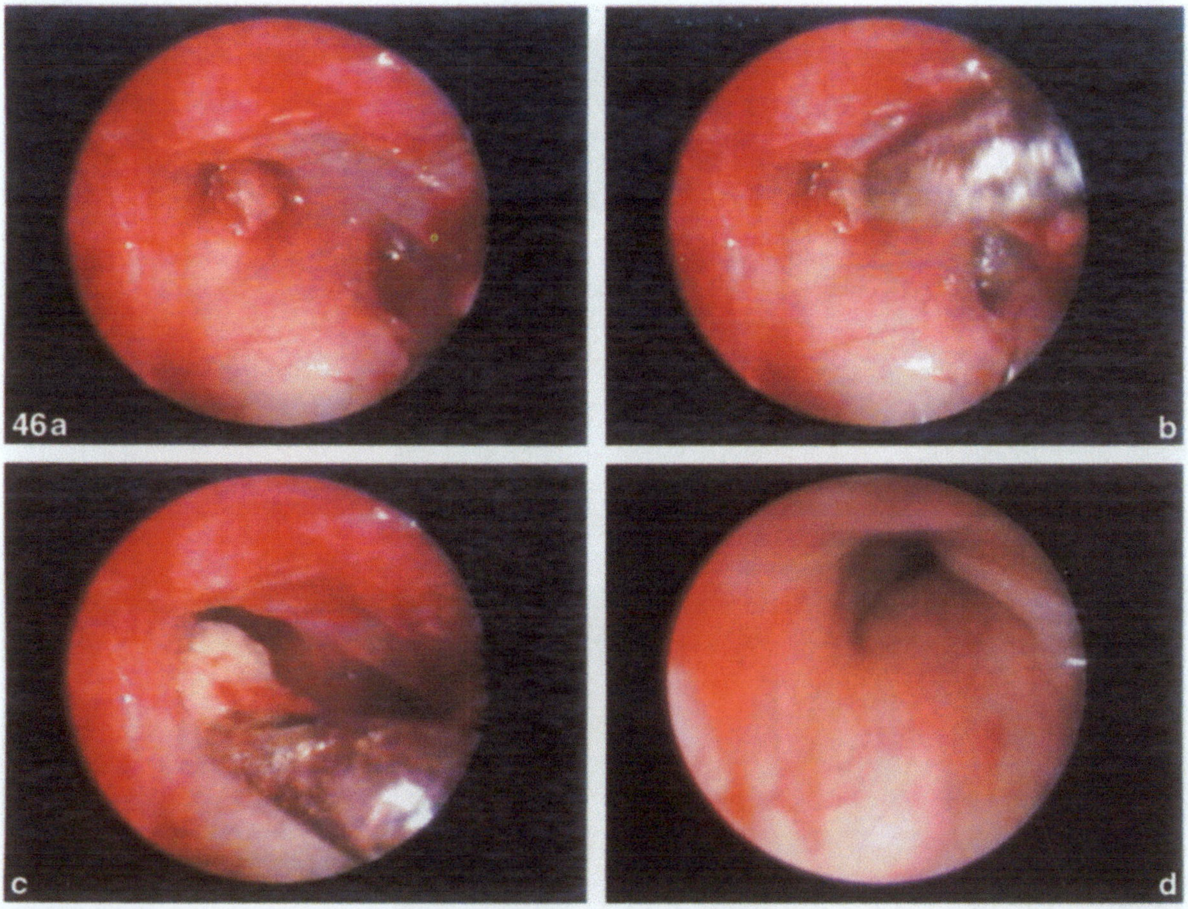

Fig. 46 a-d. Right ear: endoscopic guided surgery of protympanum (videoprint). **a** Epidermal fragment embedded in protympanum; **b, c** excision of epidermis by micro-aspiration under 0° optical system; **d** survey of protympanum, which is free of cholesteatoma

Fig. 44 a-d. Right ear: survey of epitympanum (videoprint). **a** Anterior epitympanum; **b-d** view of protympanum; **c** fistula of lateral semicircular canal

Fig. 45 a-d. Right ear: survey of protympanum (videoprint). **a, b** Protympanum: the slit corresponding to the tubal isthmus is visible at the base (0° optical system); **c** survey of tympanic cavity; **d** survey of retrotympanum; there is no epidermal residue at the sinus tympani

tubal ishthmus. The magnification obtained from the optical image allows more scrupulous checking, and even completion of eradication under endoscopic guidance if an epidermal fragment is seen (fig. 46a-d).
Inspection of retrotympanum

With a 0° system

After dissection of the cholesteatoma in the region of the windows using the operating microscope, we first insert into the tympanic cavity an optical system of 2.7 mm diameter and 0° angle of vision, coupled with the camera. Advance of the camera, held by the left hand, is monitored on the video screen. We then follow the posterior bony wall of the EAM, until the system suddenly gives a panoramic view of the internal wall of the tympanic cavity (fig. 47 a,b). One then engages in a search for any fragment left in the region of the windows.

The operator's left hand is steadied on the opera-

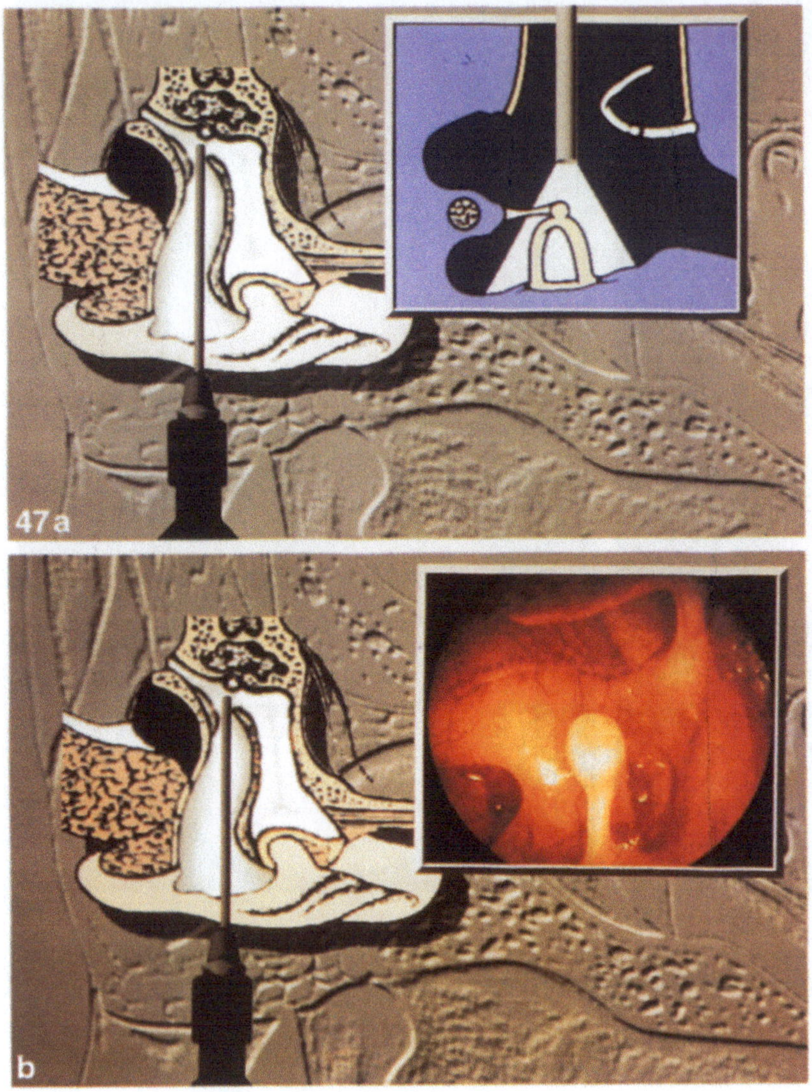

Fig. 47 a, b. Endoscopic monitoring of tympanic cavity. **a** Field of vision obtained with 0° optical system introduced into EAM; **b** endoscopic view with 0° optical system of the inner wall of the tympanic cavity (left ear)

tive towel covering the temporofacial region of the patient. This provides good stabilisation of the hand, preventing any oscillatory movements of the camera-optic couple.

The very great depth of field of the teleotoscope makes it possible to keep well away from the superstructure of the stapes (2 to 3 mm), thus avoiding any untoward contact with this ossicle. If there is major bleeding, which might possibly put a halt to this technique, small pieces of gelfoam impregnated with adrenalin are used, and left in place for 2 to 3 minutes before removal. The whitish appearance of the epidermal debris is easily identifiable in relation to the mucosa covering the bony walls.

In some cases of epidermosis, or in some very deep posterior retraction pockets, the fineness of the epidermis may sometimes make identification difficult. Excision must be performed methodically, quadrant by quadrant, always under visual control.

With 30° and 70° systems

The 0° objective is replaced by one of 30° and then of 70°, depending on the anatomic arrangement of the posterior region of the tympanic cavity. Insertion of a 70° system into the cavity of the middle ear makes preliminary training on dissection specimens absolutely essential. To familiarise ourselves with this technique, we have routinely monitored all non-cholesteatomatous tympanoplasties with 0°, 30° and 70° systems (fig. 48 a-d). The lens of the oblique optical system is orientated towards the operator, and the camera is

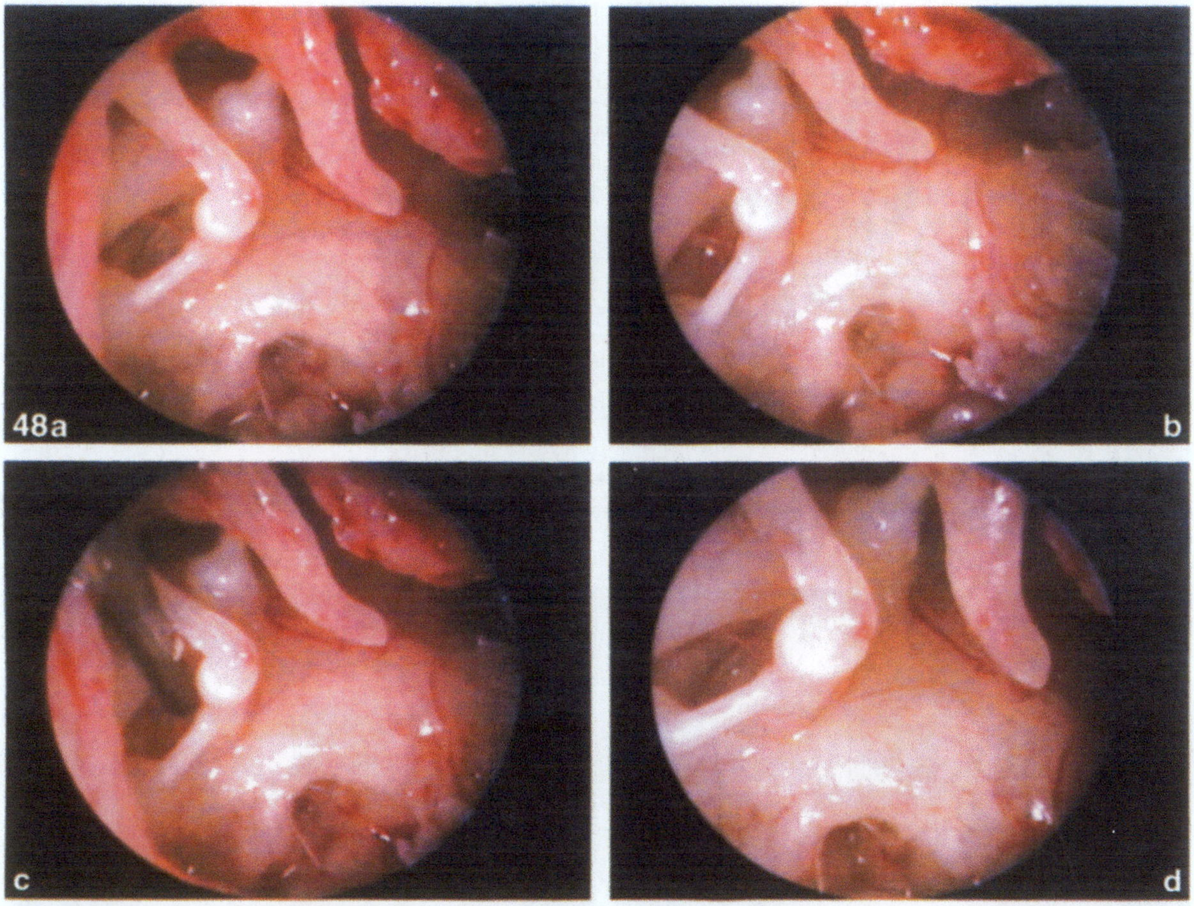

Fig. 48 a-d. Right ear: view of tympanic cavity with 0° optical system (videoprint). **a-c** Intact ossicular chain. but note appearance of long processof incus; **d** view of region of windows

fixed in good position to avoid inverted images. This assembly, always held by the left hand for a right-handed operator, allows us to follow the advancement of the lens system, previously coated with a demisting fluid, as it is guided along the posterior wall of the EAM (fig. 49).

Once the bony margin of the sulcus has been crossed, it is necessary to locate the feature constantly present, and therefore the most reliable the pyramidal eminence. The stapes may be intact or exhibit destruction of its superstructure. By circular displacement of the camera to right and left, it is possible to include the entire region of the sinus tympani in the field of vision (fig. 50 a-d):

– above, the bulge of the facial canal, but also the bony window created by the posterior tympanotomy and carved out at the expense of the facial recess

– below, the different prominences and depressions that constitute the posterior sulcus of the tympanum. With his right hand, the surgeon lowers into the retrotympanum a sucker angled at 90° which allows aspiration of accumulated blood (fig. 51 a-d). At this stage of the procedure there are several possible situations:

– either the region is free of epidermis, and the survey is concluded with assurance of complete eradication (fig. 52 a-d)

– or epidermal tissue is present.

In the latter case, ablation of the pathologic tissue will be done under video monitoring, using adapted micro-instruments, thus performing true endoscopic guided surgery (fig. 53).

Excision of cholesteatoma under endoscopic guidance

With his right hand, and under video monitorong, the surgeon progressively cleanses this region using

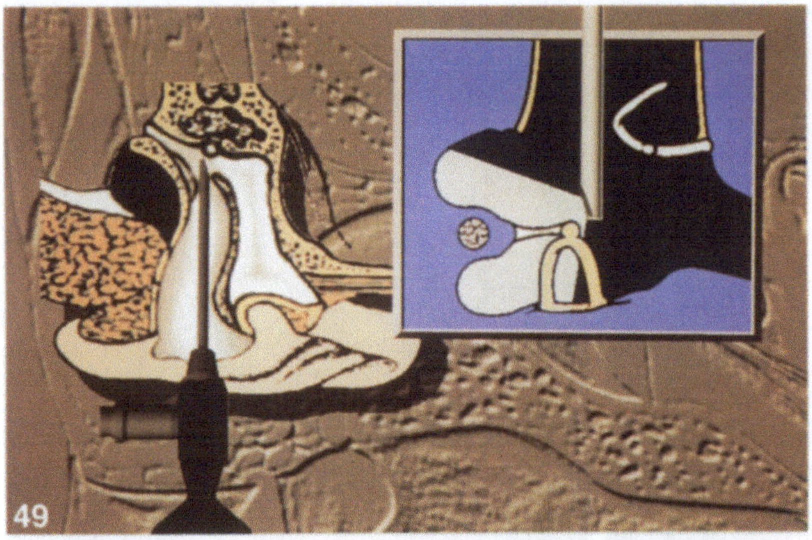

Fig. 49. Field of vision obtained with 70° optical system inserted via the EAM

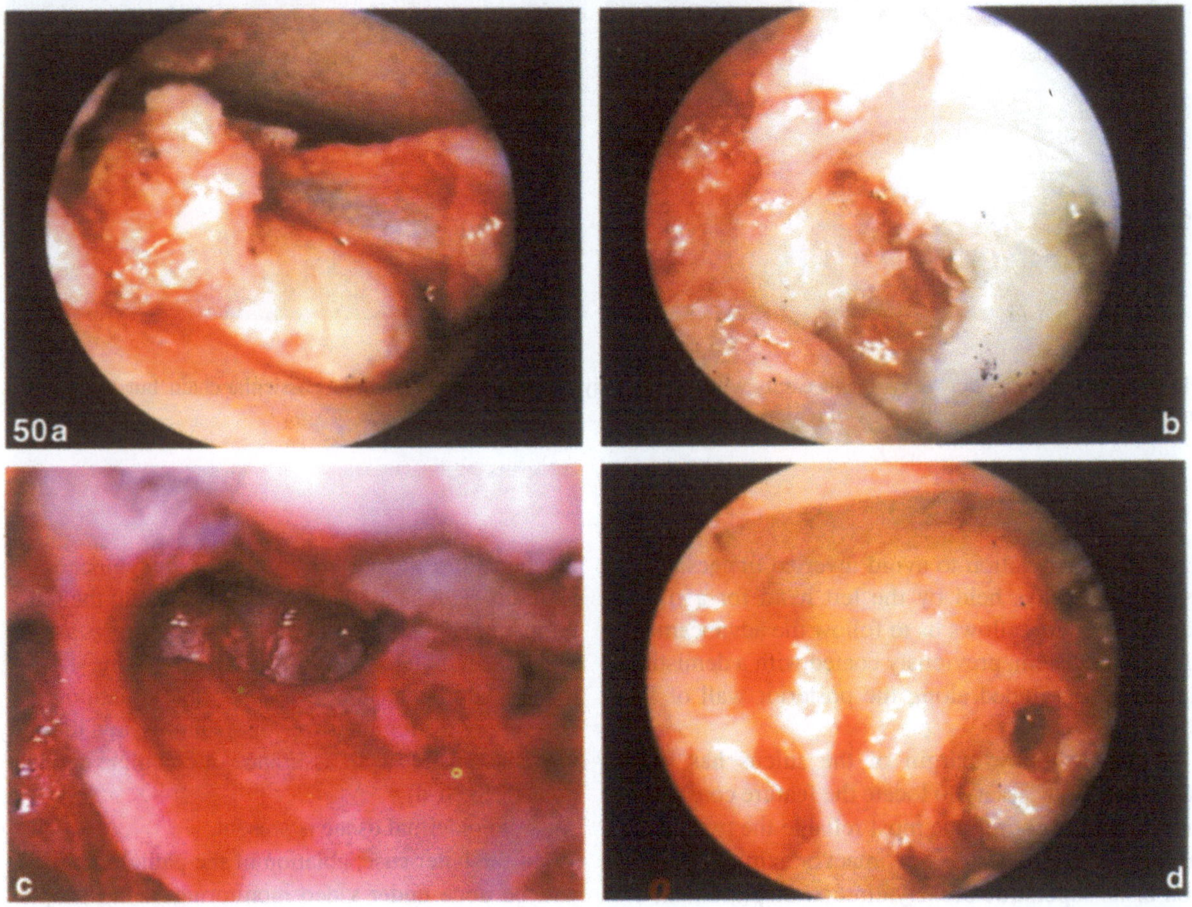

Fig. 50 a-d. Right ear: endoscopic survey of retrotympanum (videoprint). **a** Mesotympanic cholesteatoma; **b** endoscopic view of tympanic cavity after partial excision of cholesteatoma; **c** view with operating microscope, magnification x 16. The retrotymopanum cannot be seen; **d** view of retrotympanum with 70° angle optical system, showing absence of epidermal residues at sinus tympani

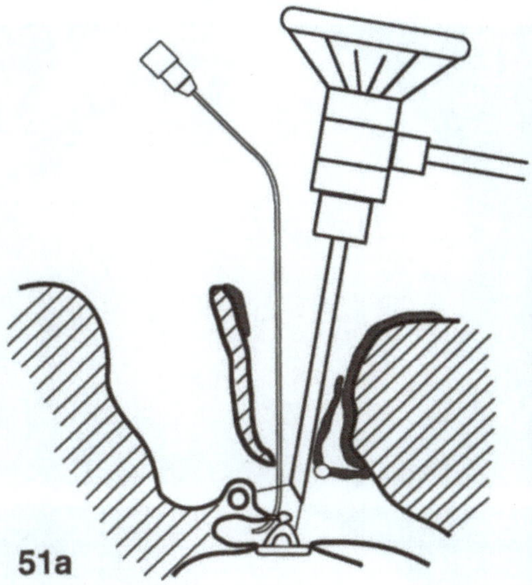

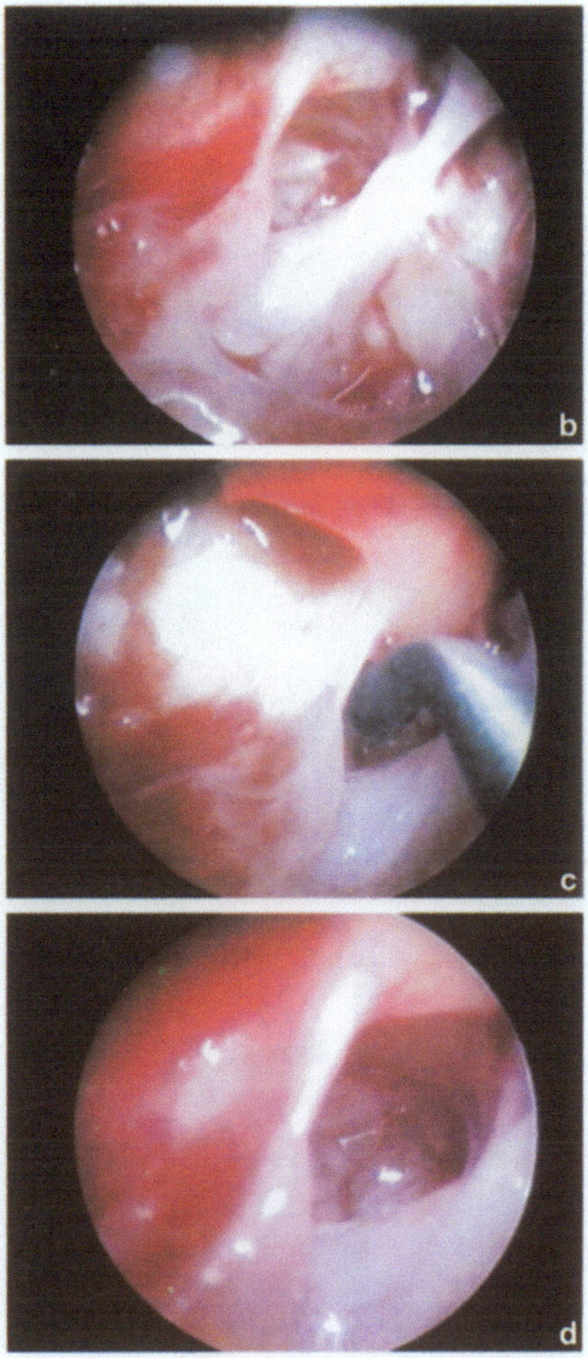

Fig. 51 a-d. Right ear: aspiration in sinus tympani under optical monitoring at angle 70° (videoprint); **a-c** Sucker angled 90° lowered into cavity; **b-d** deep sinus tympani with well-marked subiculum

micro-palettes and micro-hooks, then with suckers angled at 90° (fig. 54 a-g). Endeavoring not to withdraw the endoscope,unless soiling of the lens make this necessary, he carries out a dissection of the epidermis from wirhin outward in the direction of the posterior rim or inversely in the direction of the promontory. The fragments thus brought to a position where they are visible under the operating microscope are extracted with conventional instruments. By means of the angled aspirator, it is also possible to complete cleansing of the cavity of the sinus tympani.

Use of the 70° angled optical system, more difficult to manage than the 30° system, was indicated in 60% of our cases in conformance with the description given

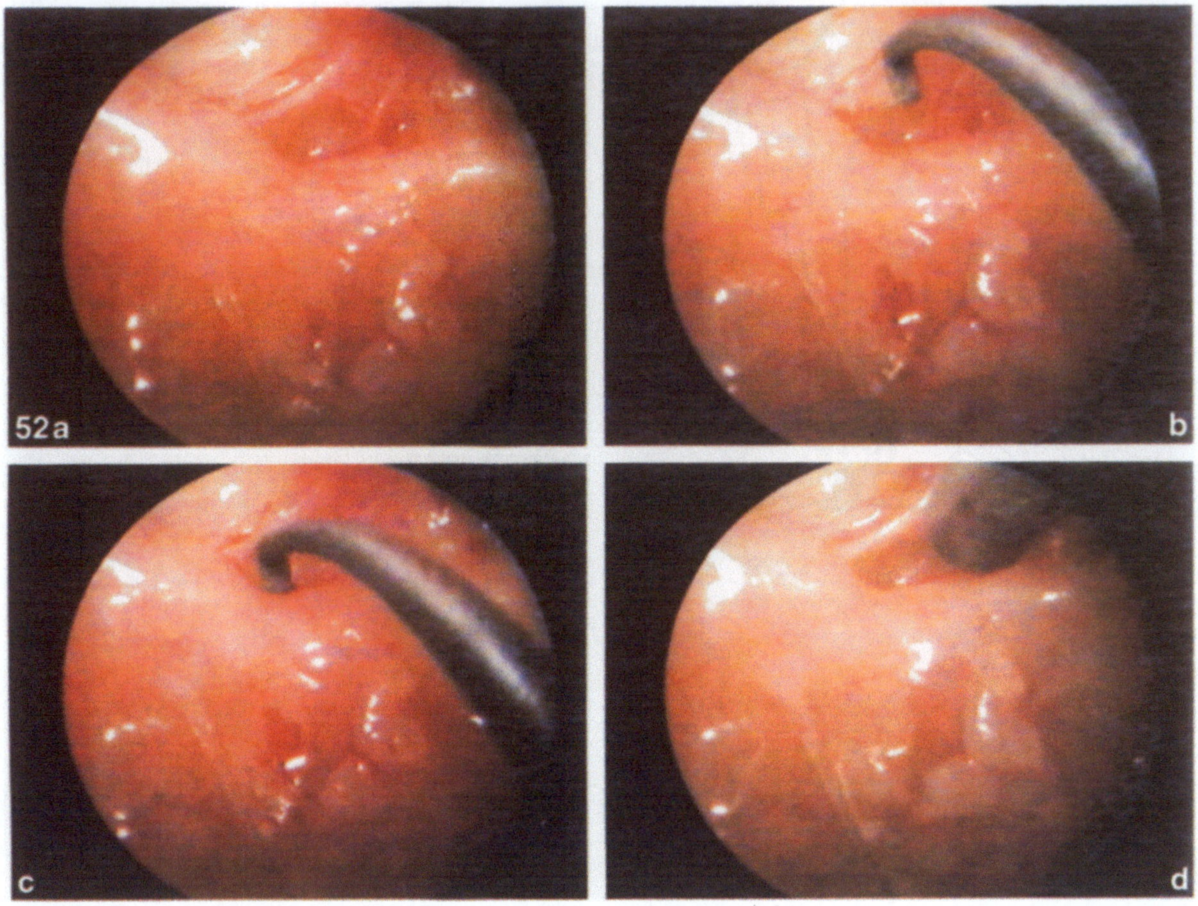

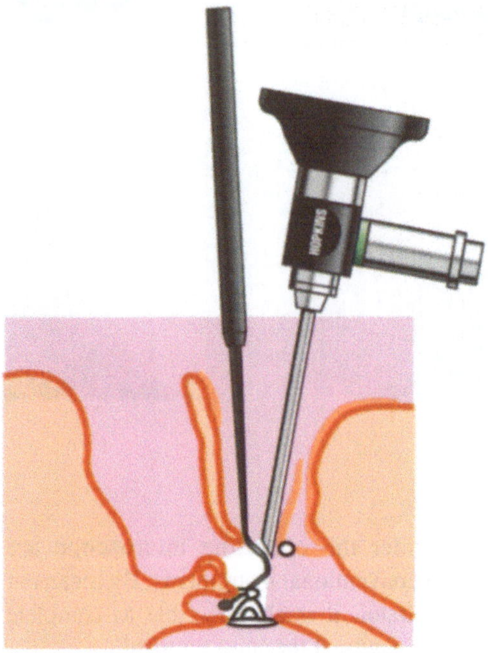

Fig. 52 a-d. Right ear: endoscopic monitoring of retrotympanum after eradication of cholesteatoma (videoprint). **a** Sinus tympani under 70° optical system (access easy); **b, c** use of micro-rugine angled at 90°; **d** micro-sucker, angled 90°, in sinus tympani

Fig. 53. Ablation of epidermal squames with micro-dissector under video monitoring

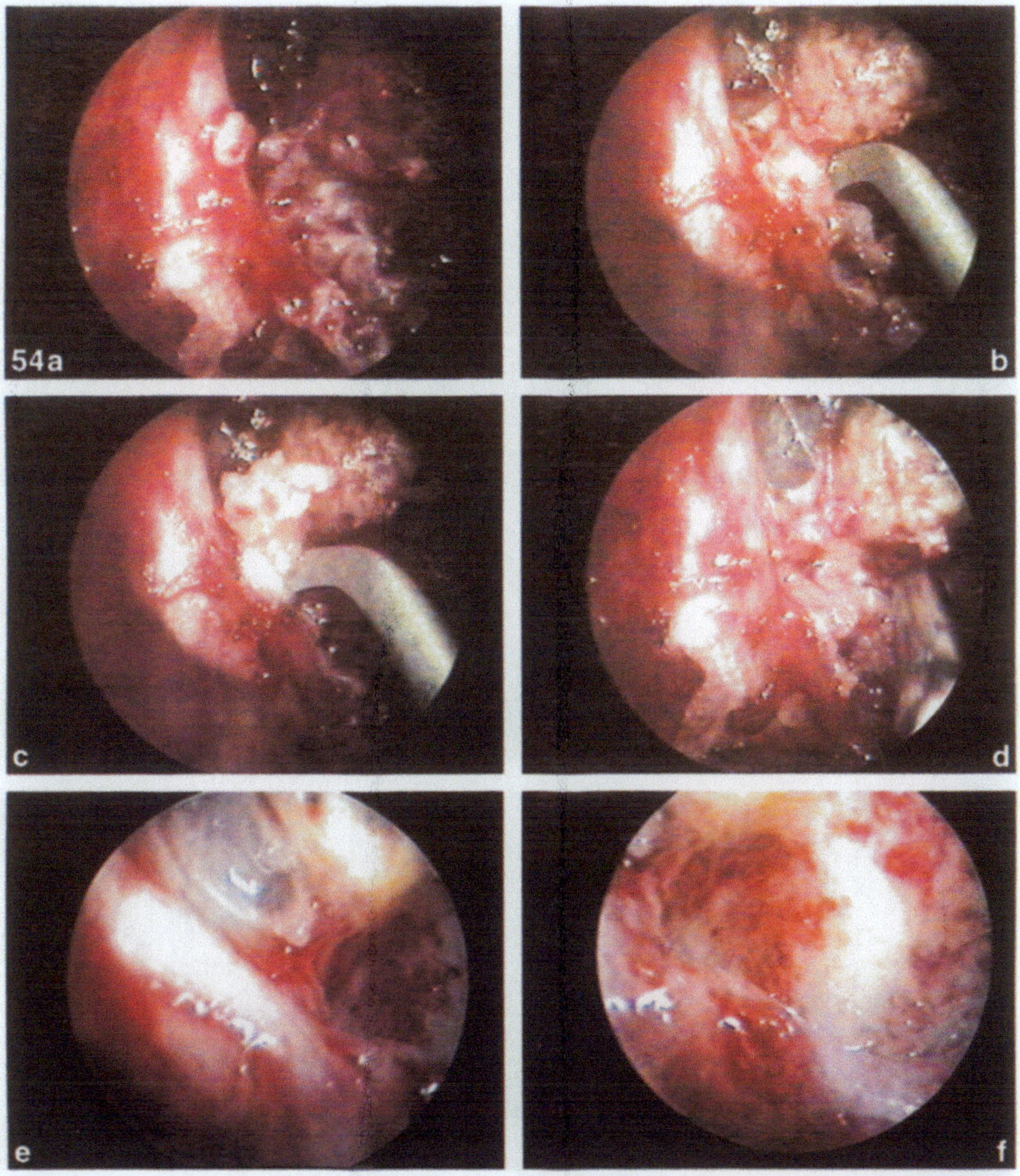

Fig. 54 a-g. Surgery of retrotympanum under video monitoring (70° optical system) (videoprint). First case: cholesteatoma in 5-year-old child. Right ear. **a** Cholesteatoma occupying entire retrotympanum; **b, c** dissection of epidermis using microdissector; **d** aspiration of epidermal fragments; **e-g** very deep posterior sulcus due to erosion by cholesteatoma

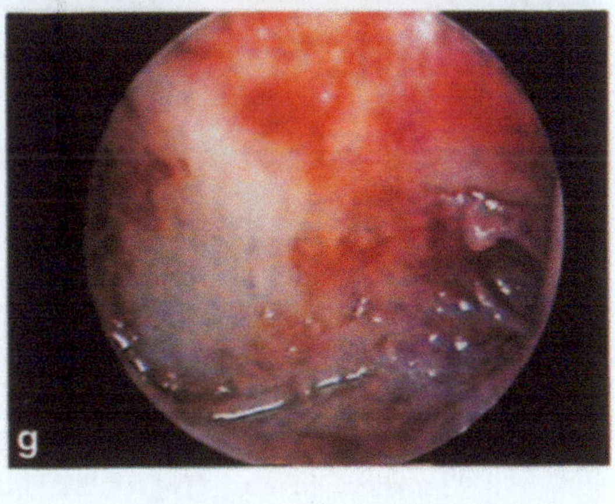

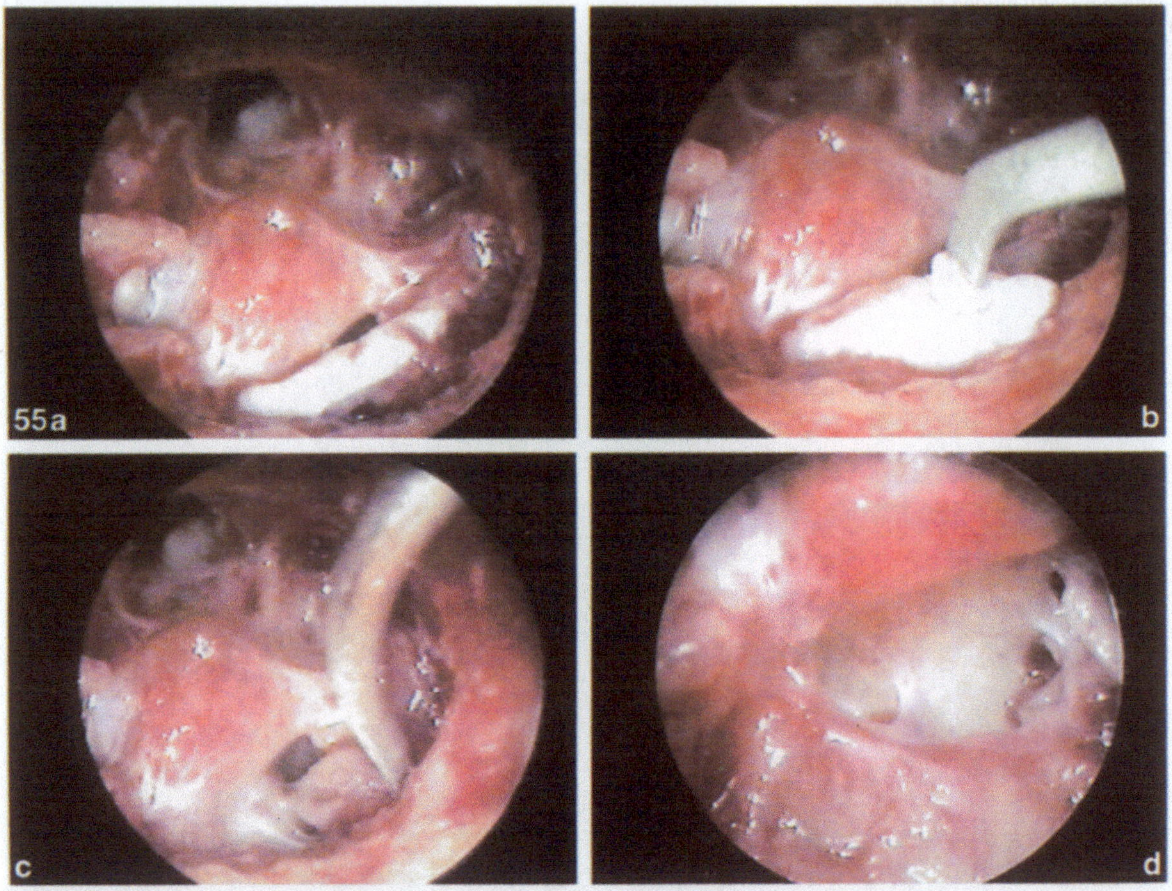
55a
b
c
d

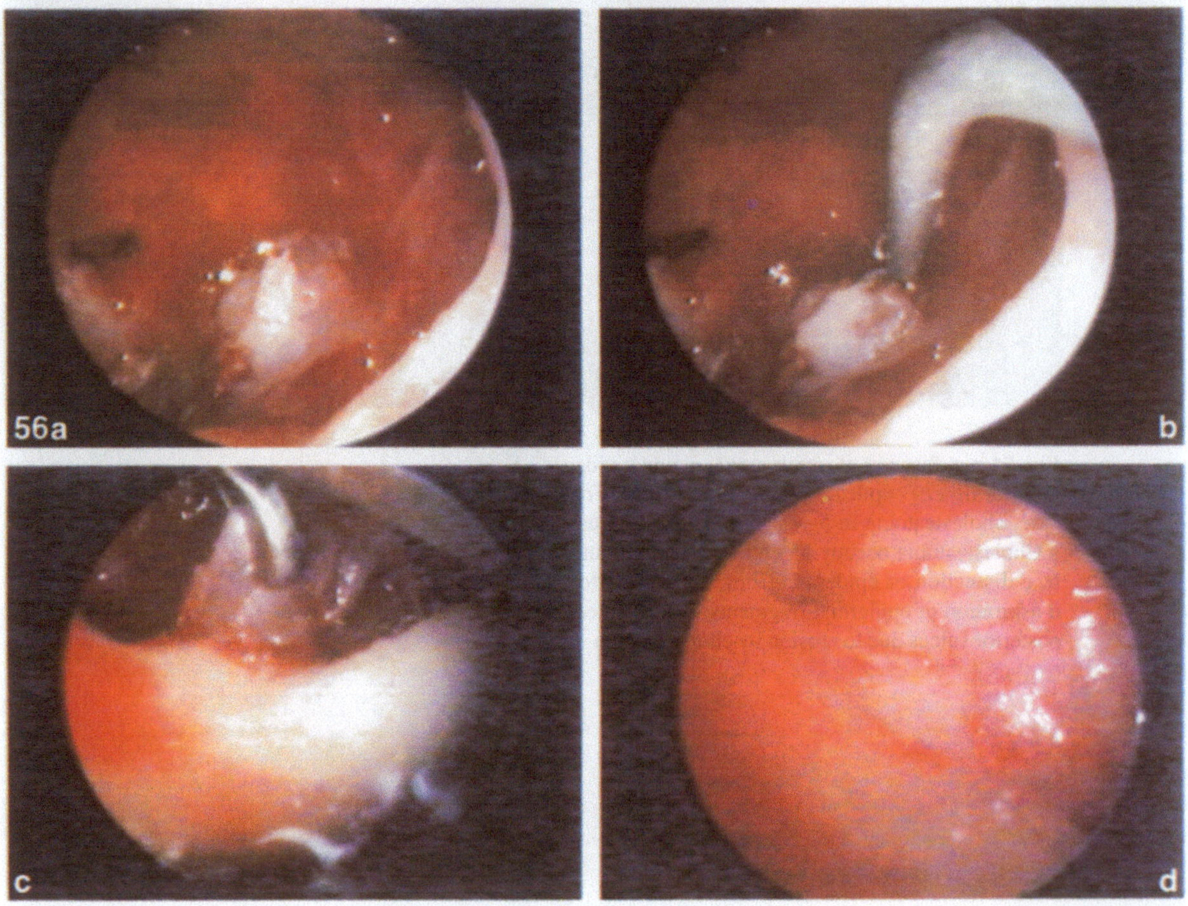
56a
b
c
d

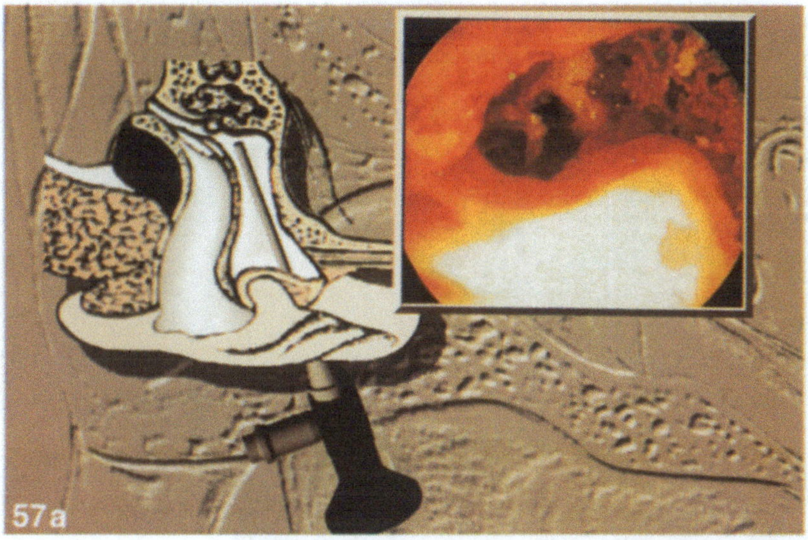

Fig. 57 a, b. Endoscopic exploration of posterior cavities using 0 and 70° systems

←

Fig. 55 a-d. Right ear: second case: epidermal spread at lower part of retrotympanum (videoprint). **a, b** Freeing with dissector angled at 90° under 0° optical system; **c** the micro-dissector progressively gathers the epidermal residues towards the promontory; **d** final survey of posterior gutter under 70° optical system

Fig. 56 a-d. Left ear:"third case: epidermosis of tympanic cavity. **a** Under 70° objective: presence of epidermal fragment at level of sinus tympani; **b, c** dissection of epidermis with micro-hook or hollow-jawed (punch) forceps; **d** final satisfactory survey of retrotympanic gutter

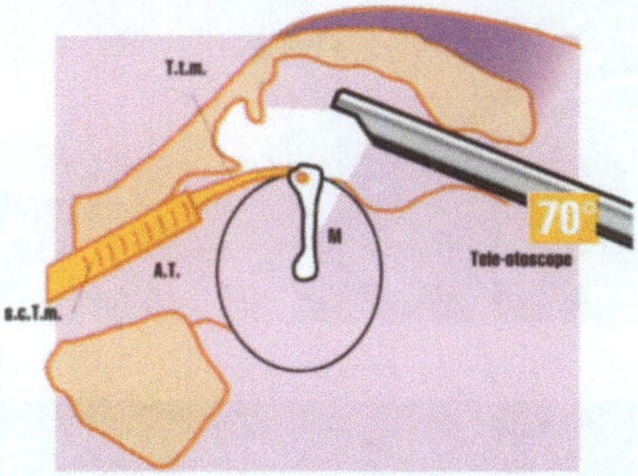

in the chapter on endoscopic anatomy (figs. 55 a-d, 56 a-d). It is now possible to couple the optical system with an operating channel to introduce an argon laser fiber of 200 or 400 π in order to vaporise the epidermal fragments and thus complete the conventional excision with micro-instruments.This new technique of guided endoscopic surgery has considerably reduced our numbers of residual cholesteatomas, since the efficiency of eradication at the first stage is greater than that possible under the operating microscope alone. However, it remains a technique supplementary to that performed with the operating microscope and is in no way a substitute for the latter. Only the management of zones of difficult access such as the retrotympanumn, epitympanum, or even the protympanum, constitute an indication for this method.

Second operative stage of closed-technique tympanoplasty

So far, we have regarded systematic surgical revision as mandatory, though its modalities are variable. The advent of endoscopic guided surgery has altered our strategy in certain cases, by allowing surgical revision through minimal cutaneous approaches under day surgery conditions.

Exploration of the posterior cavities (fig. 57)

The cutaneous approach used is a minimal reroauricular route 1 cm long situated at the retroauricular sulcus and centered on the concha, opposite the root of the helix (fig. 58). Exposure of the lining mucosa of the

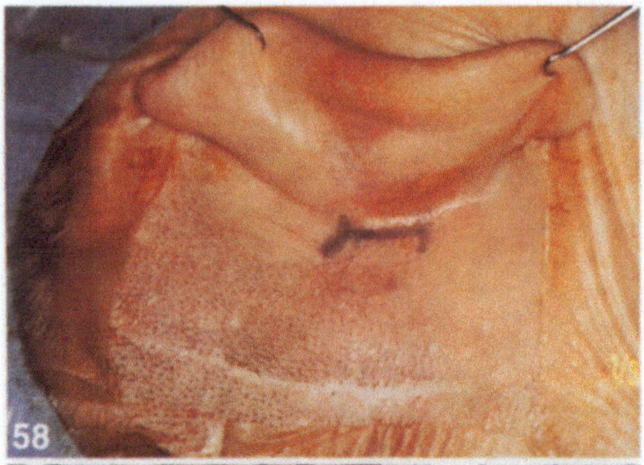

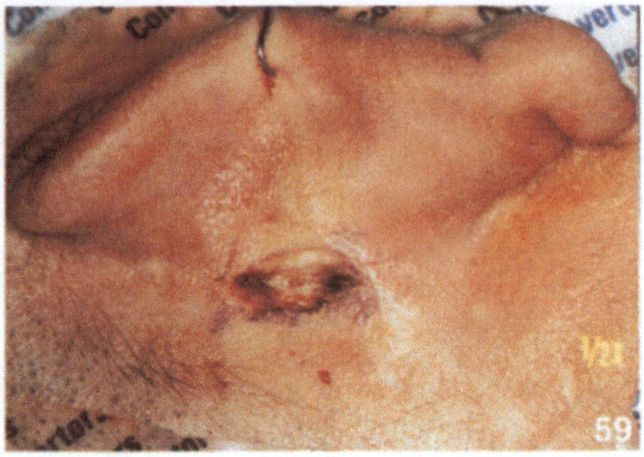

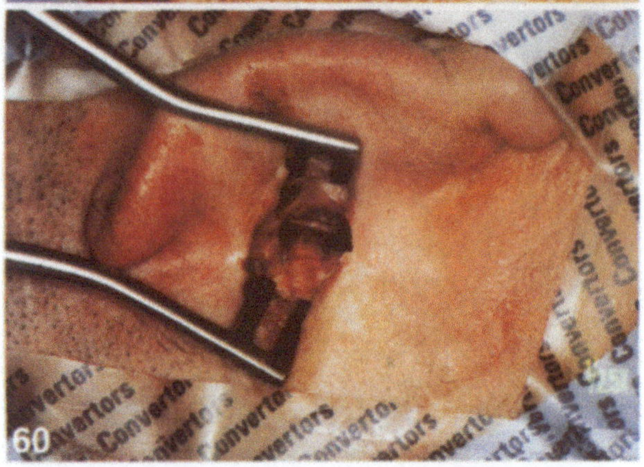

Fig. 58. Line of minimal retroauricular skin incision

Fig. 59. Section of musculoperiosteal coat

Fig. 60. Incision of mucosa lining mastoid cavity

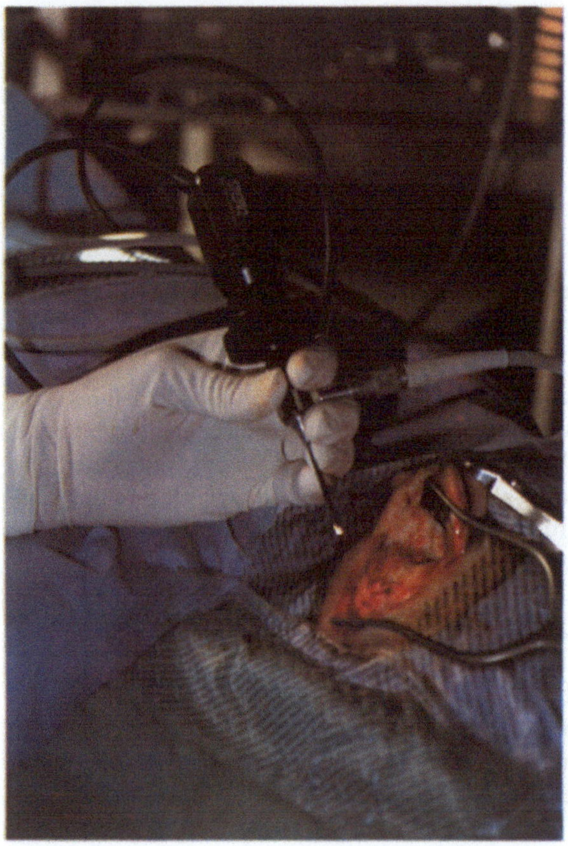

Fig. 61. Micro-camera coupled to 0°, 2.7 mm endoscope

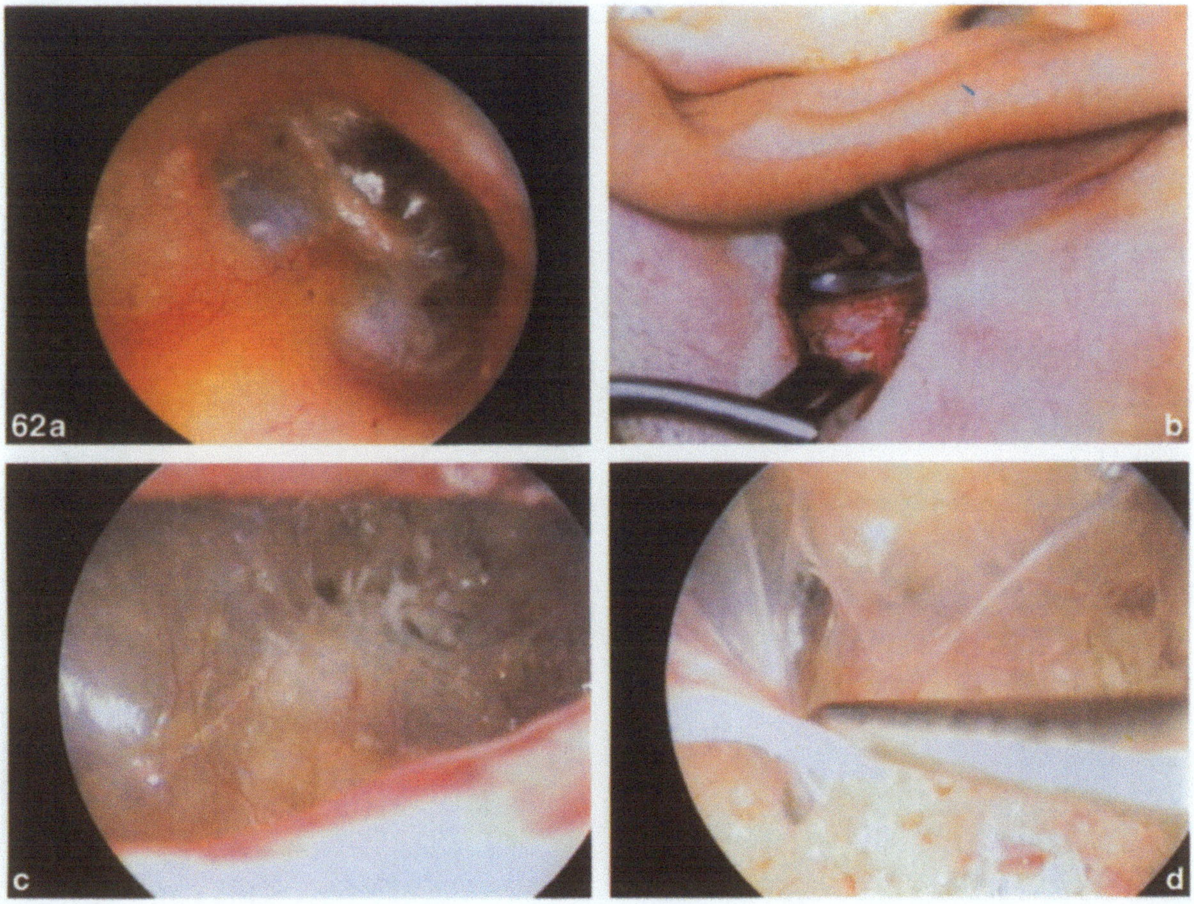

Fig. 62 a-d. Right ear: guided endoscopic monitoring of mastoido-antro-epitympanic cavity (videoprint). First case: second stage monitoring at 18 months. **a** Tympanum, appearance of graft; **b** minimal retroauricular incision; **c, d** 0° optical system used to survey mastoid cavity. There is still a mesh, which is progressively broken down

mastoid cavity is made layer by layer, moving forward. and using a No. 11 scalpel blade, while ensuring careful hemostasis with diathermy forceps (fig. 59). It is important to avoid any spilling of blood into the mastoid cavity. A clawed self-retaining retractor holds the skin edges apart (fig. 60).

Inspection of the mastoid cavity

The incision of the mucosa is performed using a scalpel with a pointed blade. The instrument nurse will have previously prepared the micro-camera equipped with a 2.7 mm endoscope of 0° angle. This assembly, held in the left hand of a right handed operator is inserted into the mastoid cavity (fig. 61). Even in the perfectly healthy ear, there is always a mastoid mesh which is broken down with micro-instruments and diathermy forceps. The lens is moved in a circle to sweep the mastoido-antro-epitympanic cavity in the direction of the tegmen antri, the posterior bony wall of the EAM, and finally the tip of the mastoid, in the search for any residual pearl (fig. 62 a-d).

If the patient is on assisted ventilation, the anesthetist may be requested to interrupt the supply of nitrous oxide responsible for misting of the lens system.

Inspection of the epitympanum

Inspection of the mastoid cavity is followed by inspection of the epitympanum. The optical system is advanced forward in the search for the bulge of the lateral semicircular canal.

It is often necessary to open several of the meshes with a retro-angled micro-dissector to permit advance of the objective, taking care not to soil its tip (fig. 63 a-d). If this does happen, it must be withdrawn from

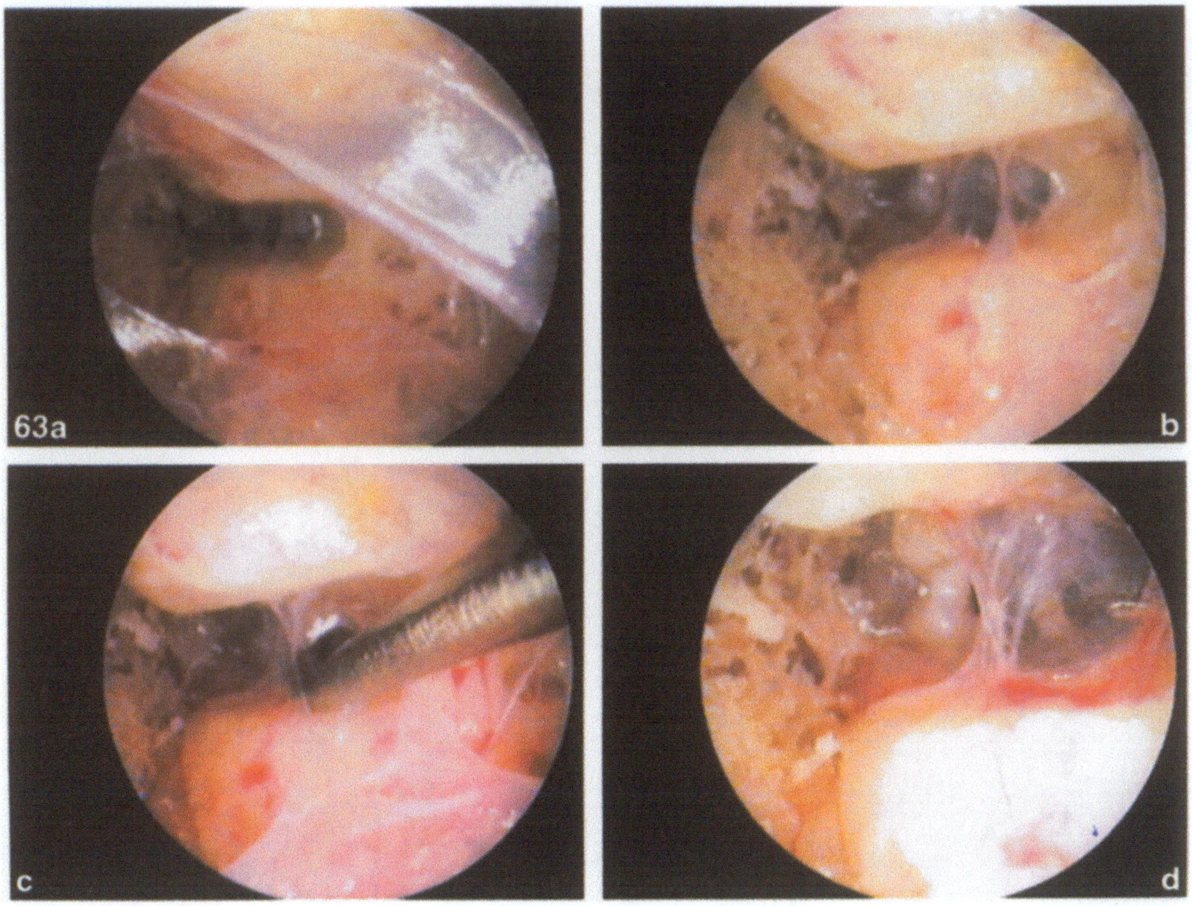

Fig. 63 a-d. Survey of epitympanum (same patient) (videoprint). **a, b** The lateral semicircular canal is located, also the window of the posterior tympanotomy; **c** partial section of mesh by micro-dissector which blocks the posterior tympanotomy window; **d** survey of anterior epitympanum. Note absence of residual cholesteatoma

the cavity, cleaned and reinserted. The exploration is pursued up to the anterior wall of the epitympanum. Thanks to this video-monitored technique, one can, in a few minutes, perform a scrupulous revision of the entirety of the mastoido-antro-attical cavities via a minimal cutaneous approach (figs, 64 a-d, 65 a-h).

A residual cholesteatoma, appearing in the form of an epidermal pearl, but also more rarelt like a splash of candle-grease, appears under the cold-light system with a characteristic pearly whiteness (fig. 66 a-d). Depending on its position, it is perfectly possible to perform ablation with the adjacent mucosa under endoscopic guidance using micro-instruments (fig. 67 a-d). Use of the argon or KTP 532 laser also allows easier vaporisation of the mucosa in the region of the pearl.

If there is a major recurrence, or if bleeding hinders the dissection, the surgeon will be compelled to enlarge the skin incision as in the classical retroauricular approach, and then proceeed to inspection under the operating microscope.

Inspection of the the tympanic cavity by the posterior route (fig. 68)

This can be performed in two ways:

– via the window of a posterior tympanotomy. This is usually obstructed by a fine membrane (fig. 69 a-e). After its ablation under vision, the wide angle of the lens system of 0° angle and 2.7 mm diameter reveals, besides the bulge of the second portion of the facial canal, the head of the stapes when this is present, but

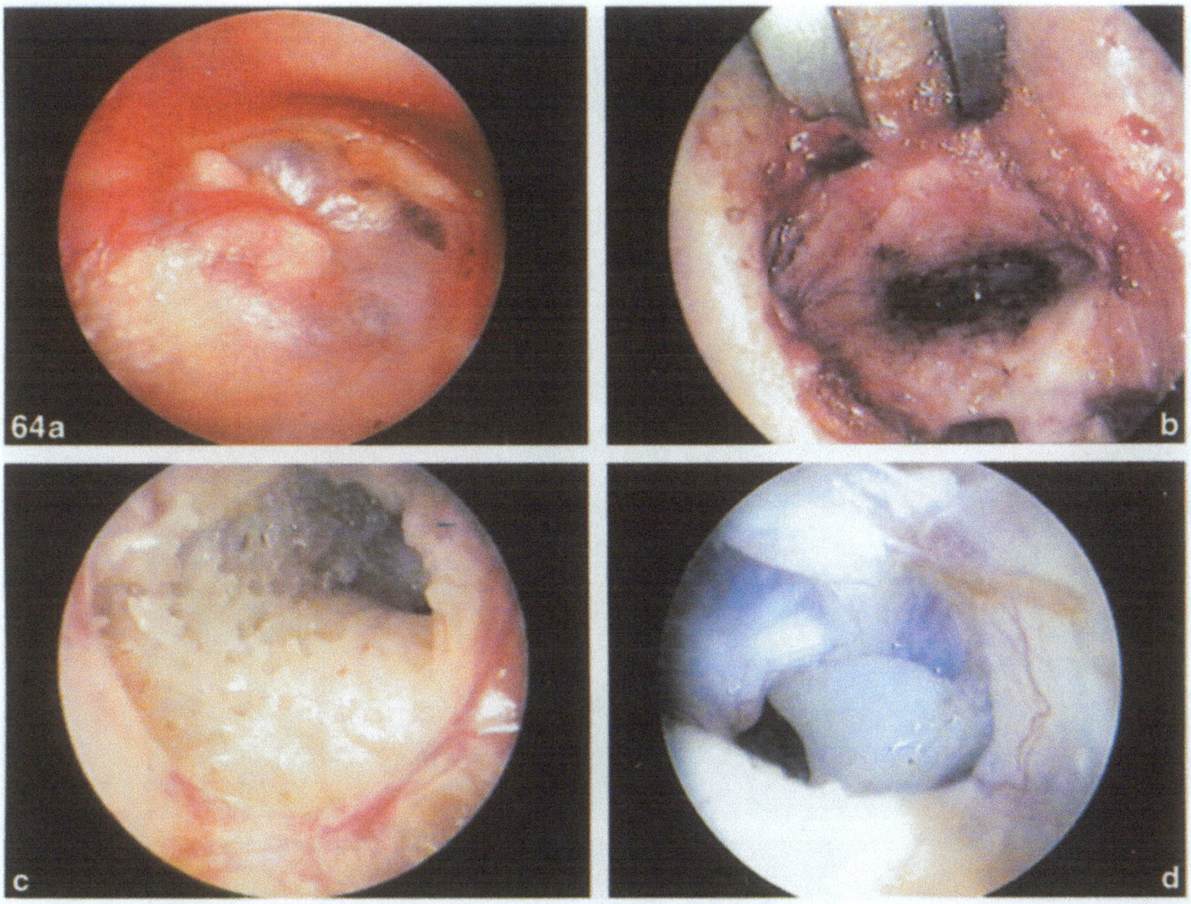

Fig. 64 a-d. Second case: right ear, second stage monitoring at 20 months (videoprint). **a** Otoscopy: tympanum, graft in order with bulge of transposition of incus performed at first stage; **b** minimal transmastoid approach; **c** survey of epitympanum (0° system): no residual pathology; **d** view with 70° system showing transposition of incus

also the outline of the semi-canal for the tensor muscle of the malleus, as well as the handle of the malleus in the event that it has been possible to preserve it;

– by the insertion into the epitympanum of 30° and 70° angle, 2.7 mm diameter systems, and then pivoting the endoscope-camera system slightly to obtain a complete view of the inner aspect of the tympanic membrane and also of the inner aspect of the tympanic cavity as far as the hypotympanum (fig. 70 a-d). The only snag by this route is failure to inspect the region of the sinus tympani.

During the first stage, and when the cholesteatona forms a sac localised to the antroattical region without extension into the sinus tympani, the probability of an epidermal inclusion at this site is extremely small. Moreover, assessment by thin CT sections through the sinus tympani can provide useful information as to the presence or absence of such an opacity. In all these cases, after careful rereading of the operative protocol. routine inspection of the retrotympanum by a transmeatal route is not essential.

We end the procedure by an ossiculoplasty made through the window of the posterior tympanotomy. The arrangements are checked by inserting a lens system (fig. 71). However, there is sometimes a spontaneous myringo-stapedopexy, which does not call for ossiculoplasty since the audiometric outcome is quite satisfactory.

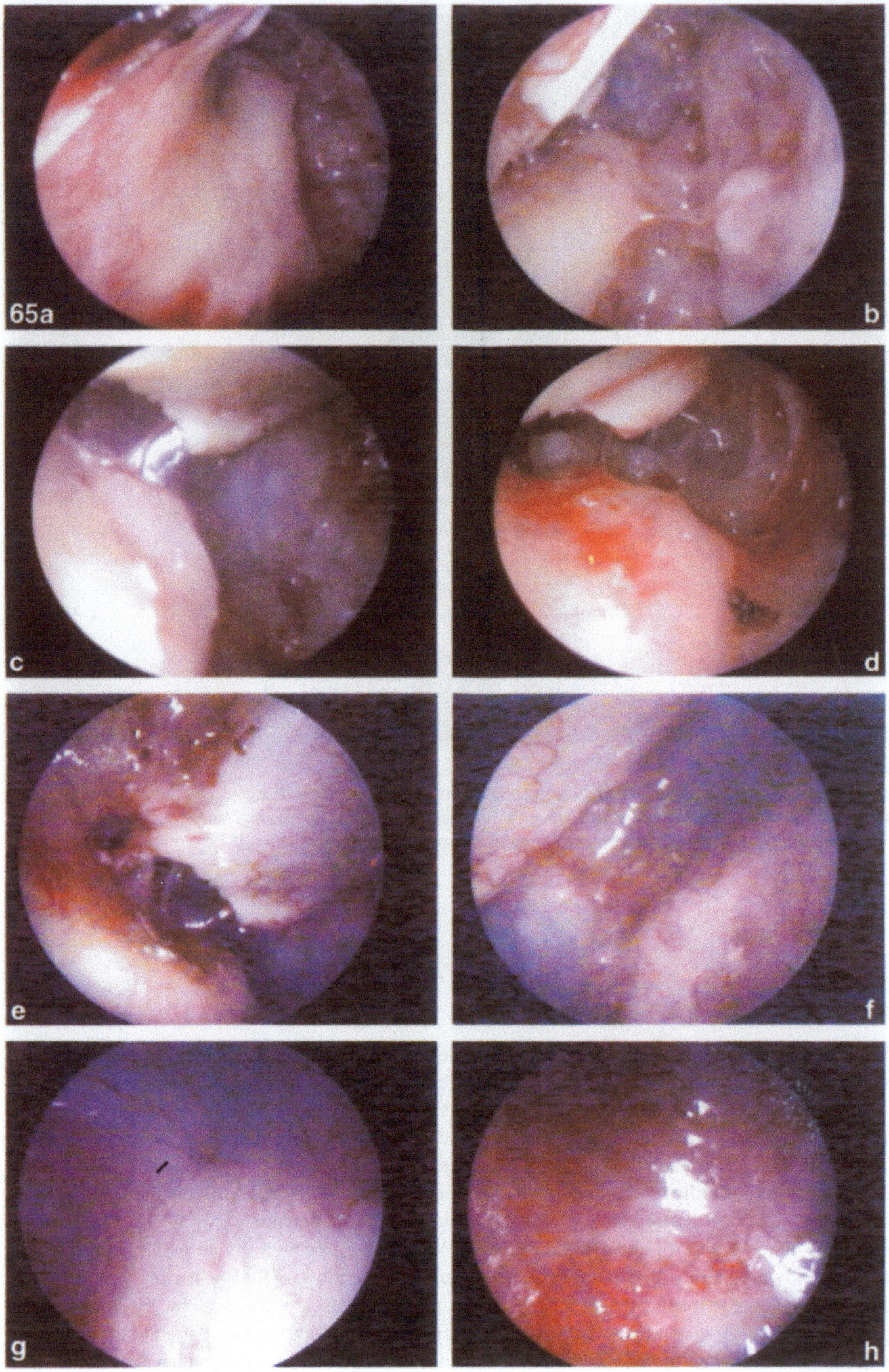
65a
b
c
d
e
f
g
h

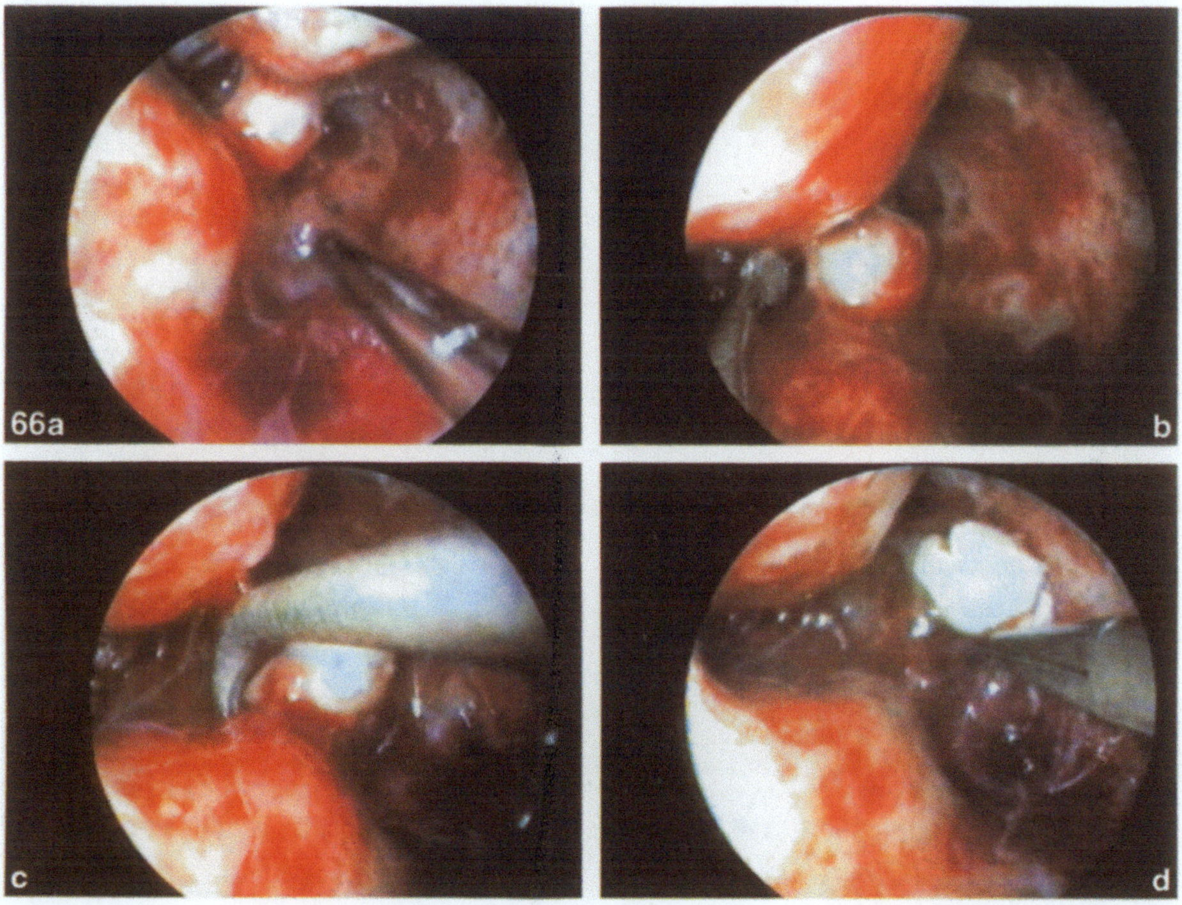

Fig. 66 a-d. Left ear: residual cholesteatoma (pearl). Minimal retroauricular skin incision. Guided endoscopic excision (videoprint). **a** Epidermal pearl on lateral semicircular canal; **b-d** dissection and ablation of pearl with adjacent mucosa under 0° lens

←

Fig. 65 a-h. Third case: left ear. Second stage monitoring at 14 months (videoprint). **a** Endoscopic view of region of lateral semicircular canal (0° system); **b** survey of anterior epitympanum. Note, above, the piece of cartilage used to reconstruct the bony defect of the EAM; **c** posterior tympanotomy window blocked by mesh; **d** after incision of mucosa. The superstructure of the stapes is visible; **e** monitoring of region of posterior tympanotomy (70° system); **f** view of anterior epitympanum and tegmen tympani; **g, h** tegmen of antrum and mastoid seen with 70° angle system

Closure of the retroauricular skin incision is performed in two layers with slowly-absorbed sutures (fig. 72).

Inspection of the tympanic cavity and retrotympanum

This is done through a transmeatal approach. An incision in made with a scalpel in the cutaneous canal at the posterior wall from 12 to 6 o'clock, thus creating a posterior meatal flap with an inferior hinge which is progressively stripped in continuity with the tympanic membrane. If the bony framework is to be reconstructed by means of a piece of cartilage, we strip this with the tympano-meatal flap. As a first stage, we perform removal of the piece of thick silastic, if this has not already been removed by the posterior route.

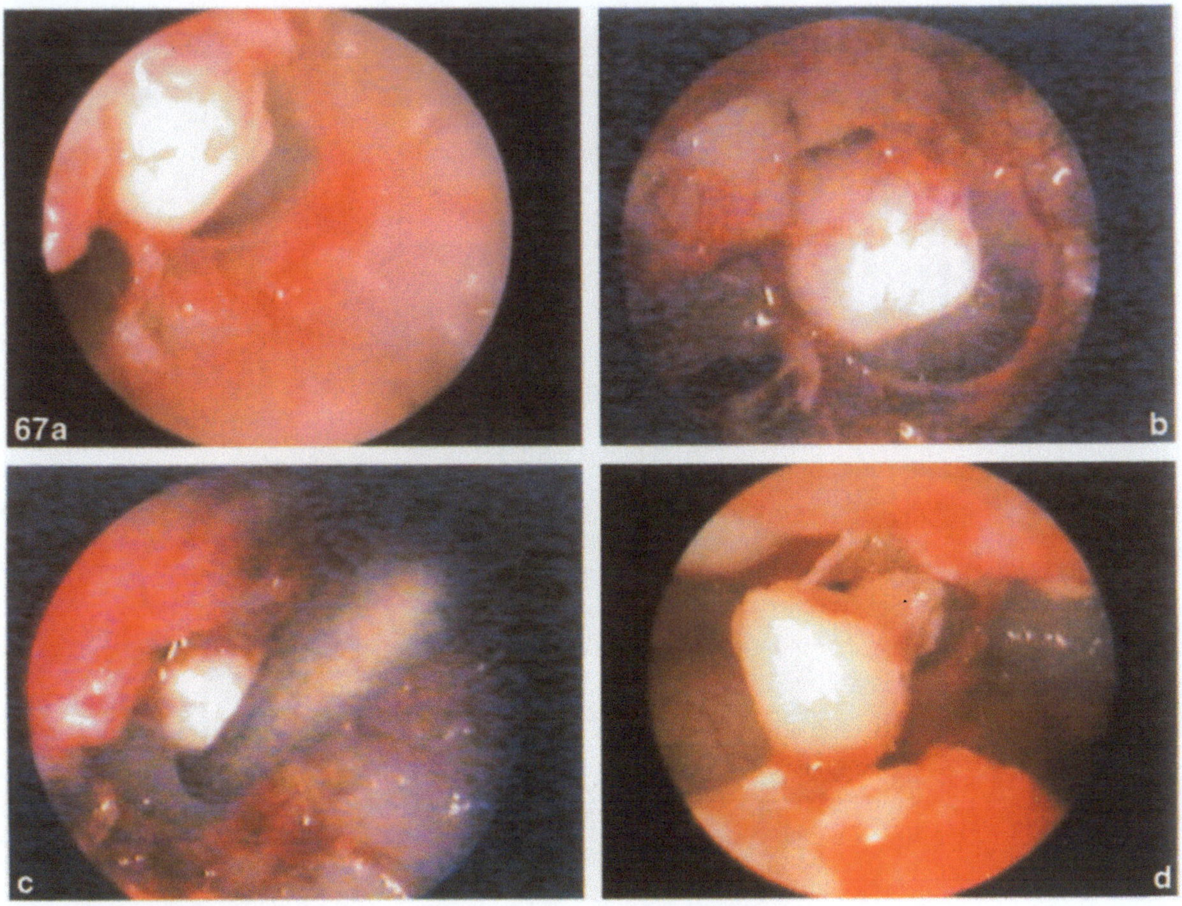

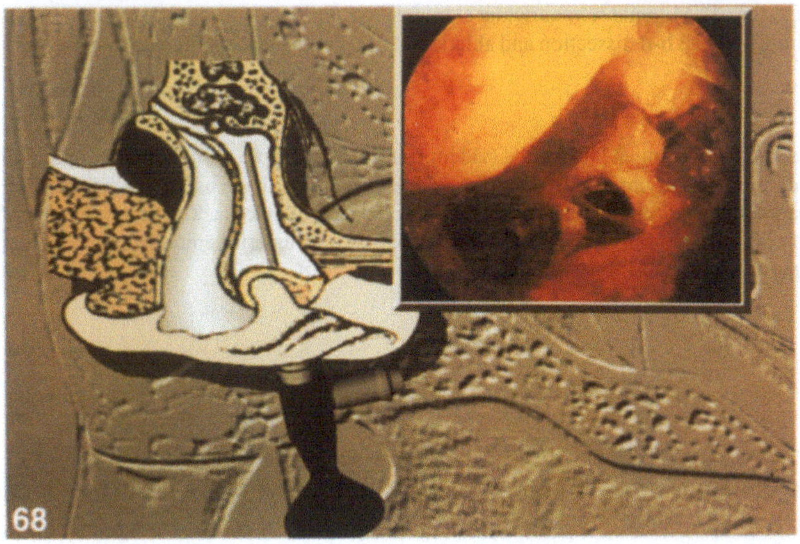

Fig. 67 a-d. Left ear: residual cholesteatoma (pearl). Retroauricular approach with minimal skin incision. **a** Epidermal pearl attached near reconstructive cartilage graft (0° lens); **b** view of pearl with 70° lens; **c, d** ablation under video monitoring

Fig. 68. Left ear: survey of tympanic cavity with 70° endoscope via posterior tympanotomy window

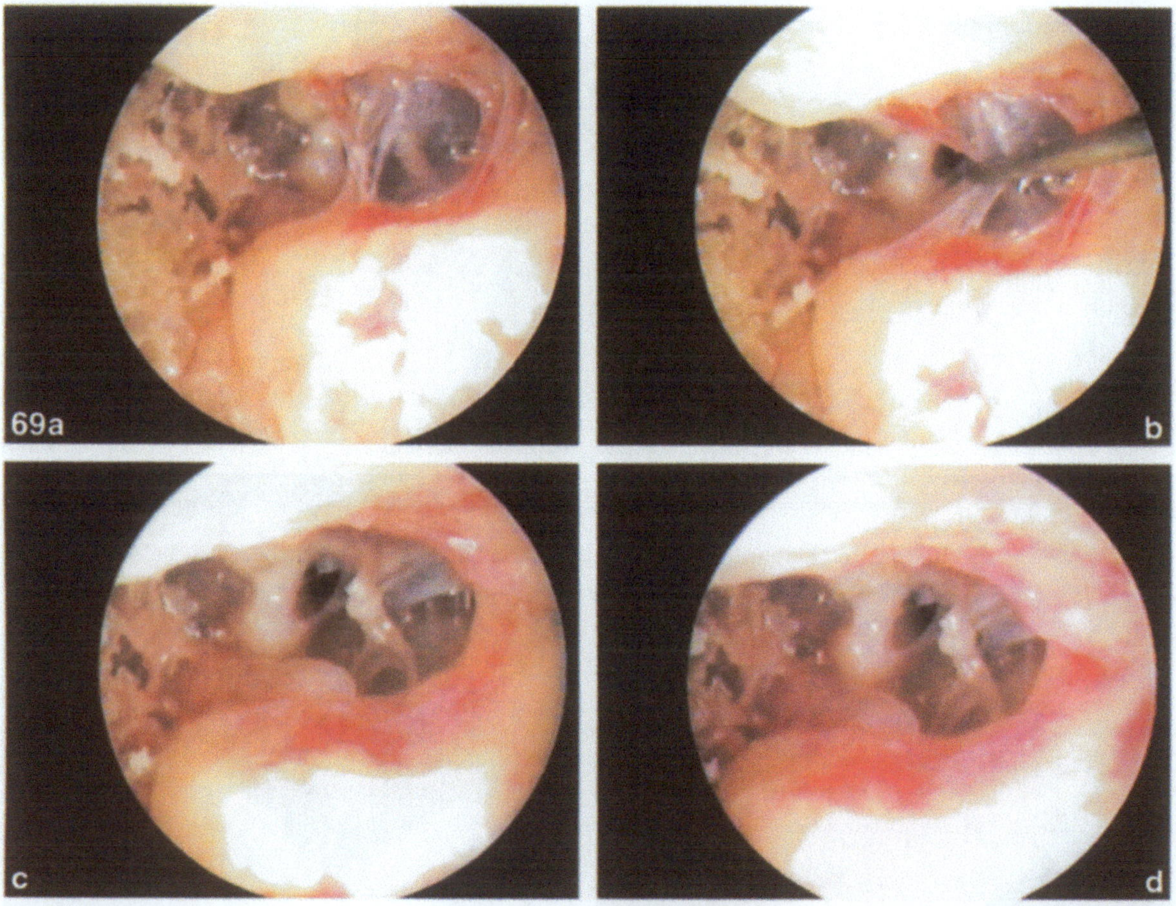

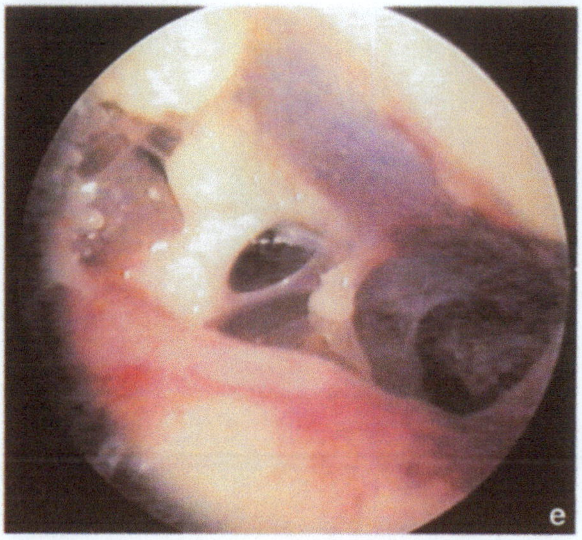

Fig. 69 a-e. Left ear: monitoring of tympanic cavity with 0° endoscope posterior tympanotomy window obstructed by fine mesh. **b** Breaking down of mesh with micro-hook; **d** angle of vision obtained on handle of malleus and stapes; facial nerve exposed; **e** view of tympanic cavity with 70° lens. There is a spontaneous myringo-stapedopexy

Inspection of the tympanic cavity

Exploration of the tympanic cavity begins with forward reflection of the tympano-meatal flap. Held in the left hand, the microcamera with its 0°, 2.7 mm endoscope, is introduced.and its progress followed on the video monitor screen placed opposite the operator.

The objective, having entered the tympanic cavity, rapidly sweeps round the medial wall, the protympanic region, the hypotympanum and the windows in the

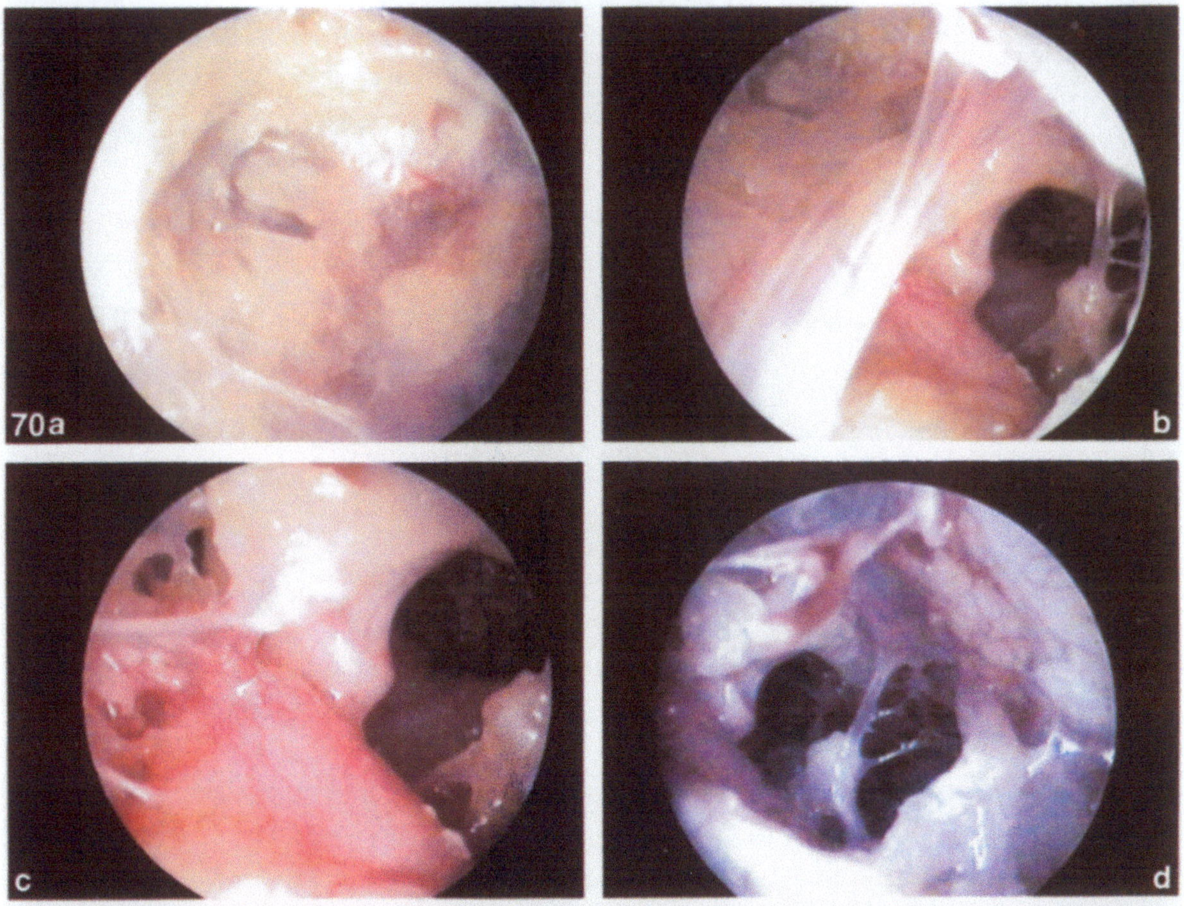

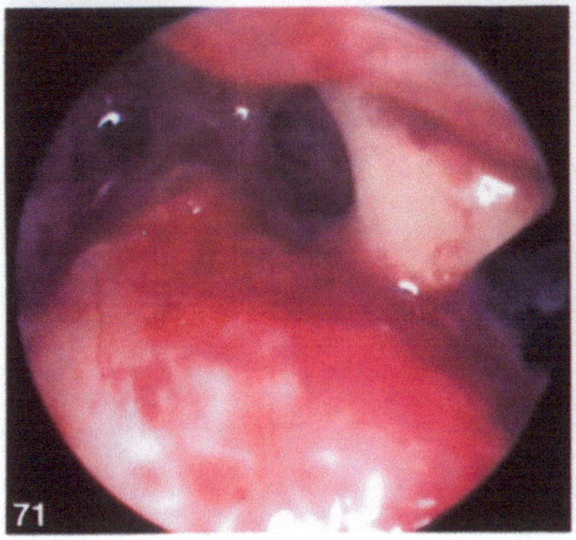

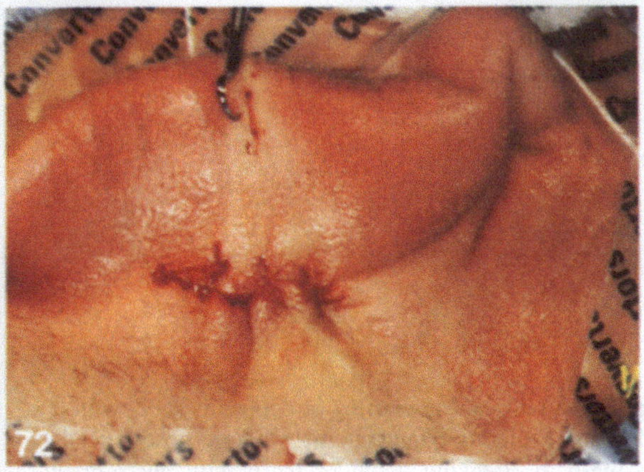

Fig. 70 a-d. Endoscopic monitoring of posterior cavities under 0° and 70° angles by a minimal posterior cutaneous approach (videoprint). **a** Survey of anterior region of epitympanum; **b, c** survey of tympanic cavity; **d** view obtained with 70° angle optical system through posterior tympanotomy window

Fig. 71. Right ear: checking of ossiculoplasty (incus) after having dressed the EAM (videoprint)

Fig. 72. Closure of minimal retroauricular skin incision (slowly absorbed sutures)

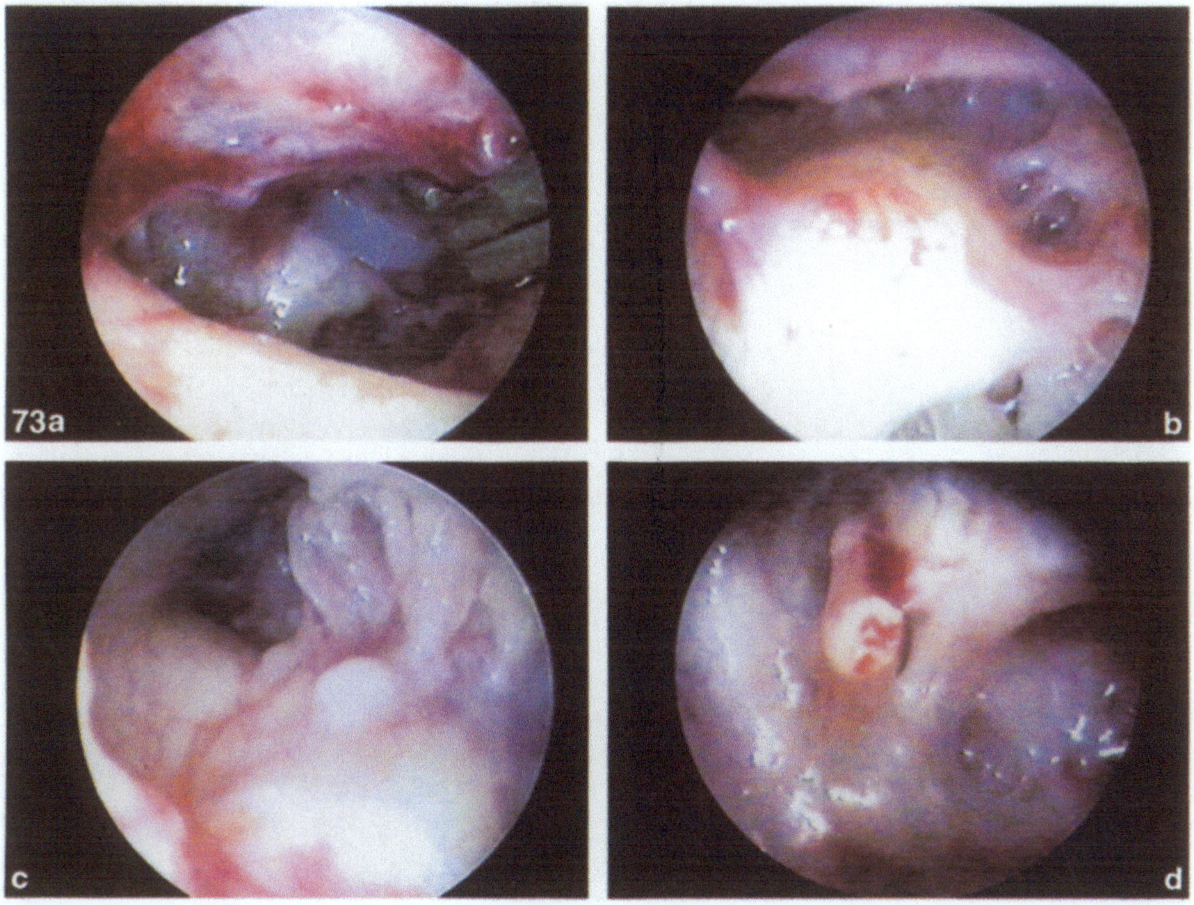

Fig. 73 a-d. Right ear: monitoring of tympanic cavity via transmeatal approach (videopriont). **a** Ablation with micro-forceps of silastic inserted at first operative stage; **b, c** inspection of hypotympanum and protympanum under 0° optical system; **d** monitoring of retrotympanum under 70° optic; no residual pathology

search for a residual cholesteatomatous pearl (fig. 73 a-d). The lens system is then withdrawn and replaced with one of 70° angle. With the end of the lens turned towards the operator and the camera still held by the left hand, the surgeon finds his orientation by identifying the posterior wall of the bony EAM up to its entry into the tympanic cavity, seeking the prominence of the pyramidal eminence (cf description of first stage) (fig. 73d), During the second stage of inspection, we use this lens system only in cases of invasion of the sinus tympani by a cholesteatoma at the first stage, and especially in the presence of epidermosis (fig. 74 a-d). While CT examination may furnish the operator with information on the state of the sinus tympani, this is in no way a substitute for endoscopic monitoring, which must be a routine for all cholesteatomas, encapsulated or not, invading the retrotymopanum at the first stage of eradication by closed or open technique.

If there is a pearl or epidermal residue (fig. 75 a-c), excision is performed by combining excision under the operating microscope with that under endoscopy, depending on the site of the recurrence (fig. 76 a-d).

Ossiculoplasty

This is usually performed by the transmeatal route under the operating microscope. The completed ossicular montage is always monitored by the introduction of a 0° system into the tympanic cavity (fig. 77), and by way of a posterior tympanotomy after packing the meatus (fig. 78).

The tympano-meatal flap is turned down. In some cases, if a retraction pocket has recurred, the posterior superior region of the tympanum is reinforced with a thin chip of cartilage based on the bony meatus and held in place with fibrin glue. The EAM is gauged with a silastic roll filled with gelfoam pellets (fig. 79), which is withdrawn on the 8th postoperative day.

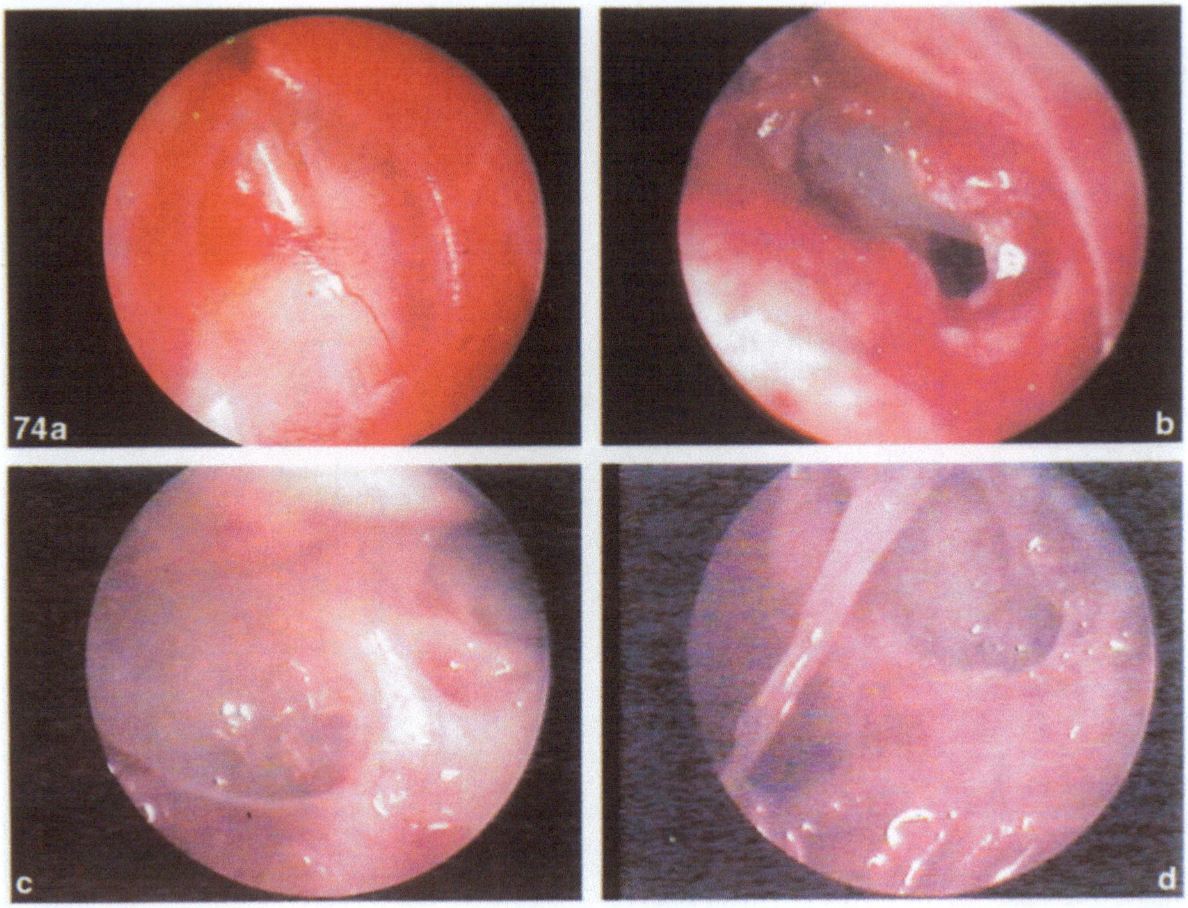

Fig. 74 a-d. Right ear: monitoring of tympanic cavity; second stage monitoring at 10 month after the first procedure (see fig 54 a-g). Child five year's old (videoprint). **a** Eardrum appearance; **b** thick silastic inserted in the tympanic cavity; **c-d** monitoring of retrotympanum under 70° optic: no residual pathology

Monitoring of the tympanic cavity by the myringotomy technique

In some cases, where the ossicular chain is intact, the approach through the conduit may be replaced by a simple myringotomy. The incision is radial, in the posteroinferior quadrant. The introduction of optical systems of 0°, 30° and 70° angles allows a precise survey (fig. 80a-d). Secondary healing of the membrane usually takes place satisfactorily. We do not favor the use of systems of less than 2.7 mm diameter since the image obtained is of poor quality.

Surgery of retraction pockets

The surgery of tympanic reinforcement is applied to localised "dangerous" invaginations, since these have either become unstable at the epidermal level or appear as marginal in relation to the bony ring. Lastly, they are nearly always adherent to the incudo-stapedial region, and so responsible for lysis, and to the region of the facial recess.

Posterior and posterosuperior invaginations (fig. 81)

The cutaneous access route is posterior, without antrotomy, but with section of the posterior cutaneous lining of the EAM. After constructing a posterior meatal flap, dissection of the epidermal pouch under the operating microscope is begun in the usual manner, step by step. The pouch is freed from the ossicular structures (long process of the incus, stapes) in atraumatic fashion, taking care not to tear it. This fine epidermis, devoid of lamina propria, is only too readily

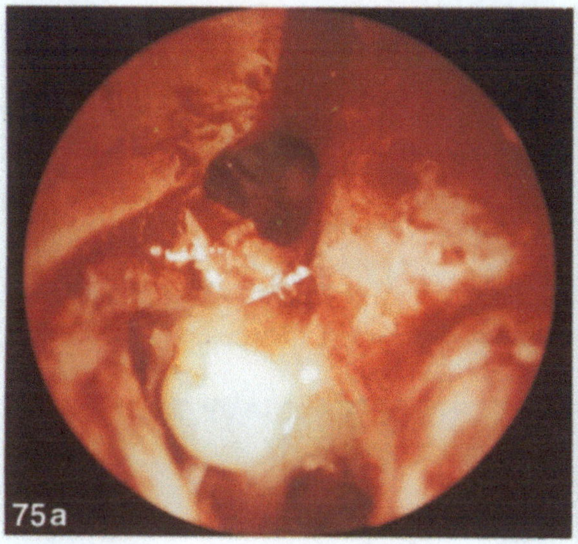

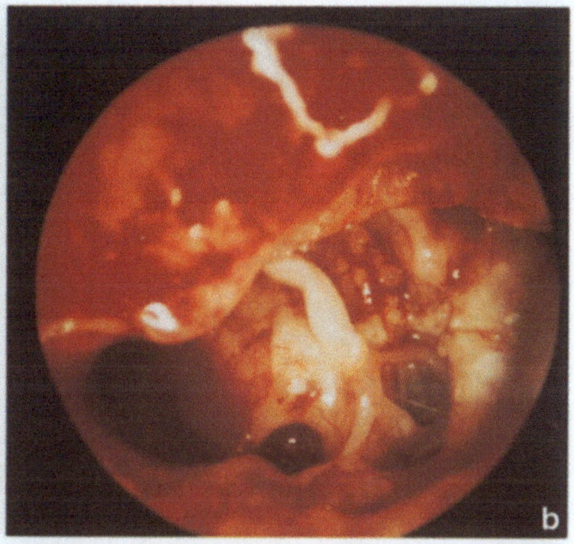

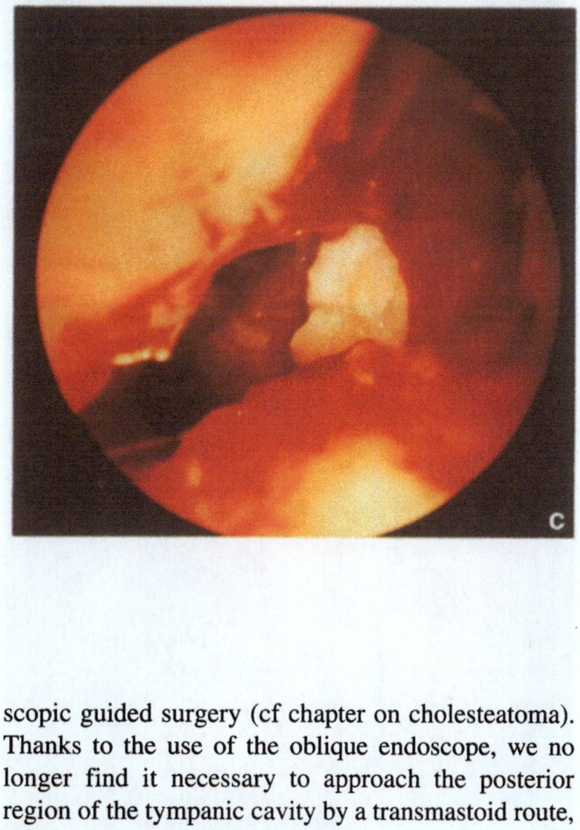

Fig. 75 a-c. Different appearances of residual cholesteatomas observed. **a** Right ear: totally circumscribed pearl covering superstructure of stapes; **b** left ear: epidermal flake at stapes; **c** left ear: unencapsulated epidermal fragment enclosing stapes

ruptured during stripping or by the cannula of the sucker. When the pocket is deeply invaginated in the direction of the facial recess and the sinus tympani region, its excision has unfortunately to be carried out blindly.

If there is rupture of the invaginated pocket, or excessive retraction of the latter, we use an endoscope to inspect the retrotympanum (fig. 82 a-d). With optical systems of 30° and 70° and under video monitoring, any epidermal fragment that may have been overlooked is sought, There are two possibilities:

– the excision has been total and is confirmed by endoscopic monitoring

– an epidermal fragment remains, requiring endoscopic guided surgery (cf chapter on cholesteatoma). Thanks to the use of the oblique endoscope, we no longer find it necessary to approach the posterior region of the tympanic cavity by a transmastoid route, through a posterior tympanotomy.

Epitympanic invaginations

When these are limited, it may sometimes be beneficial to perform transmeatal endoscopic survey using 0° and 30° optical systems to monitor the quality of the excision of the epidermal pocket; more rarely, they require endoscopic guided surgery (fig. 83a-h), When the pouch is large and extends beyond the incudo-mallear

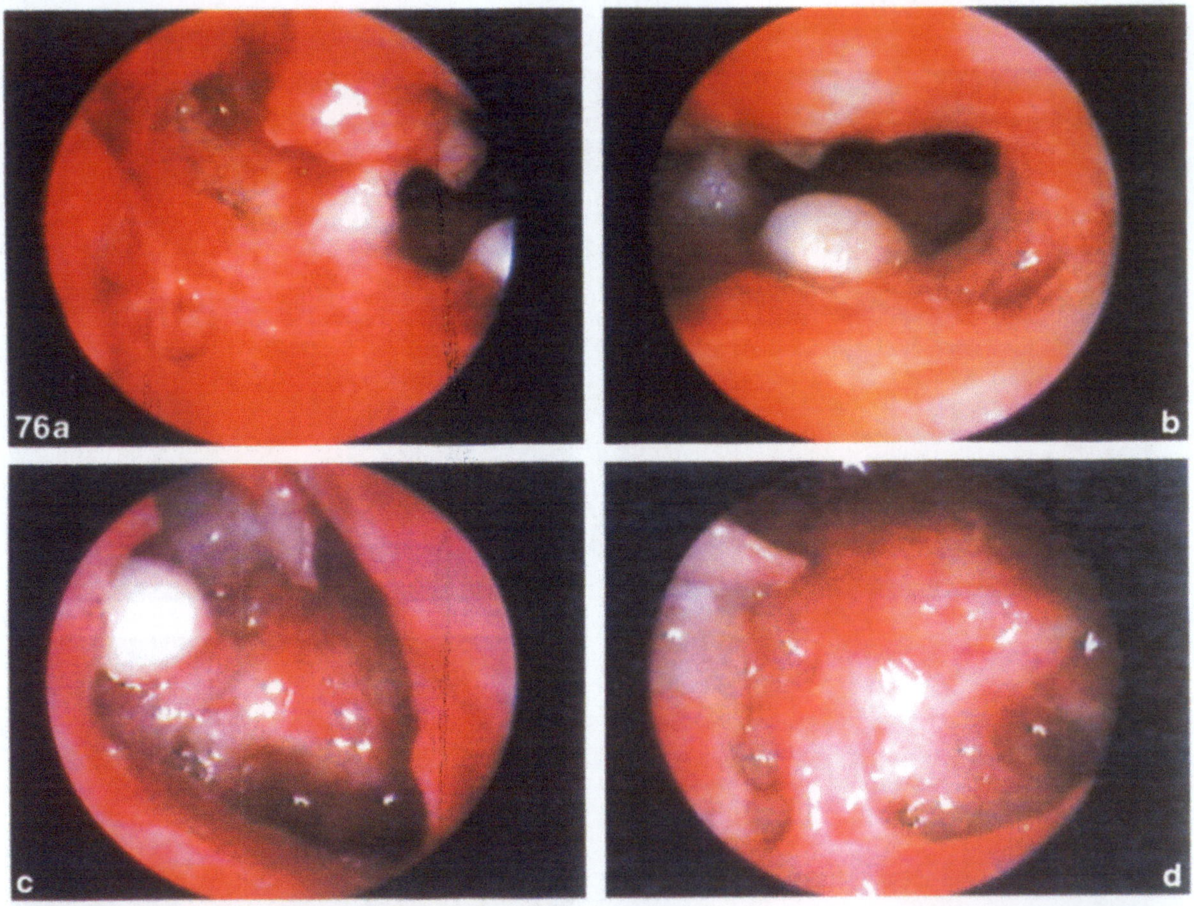

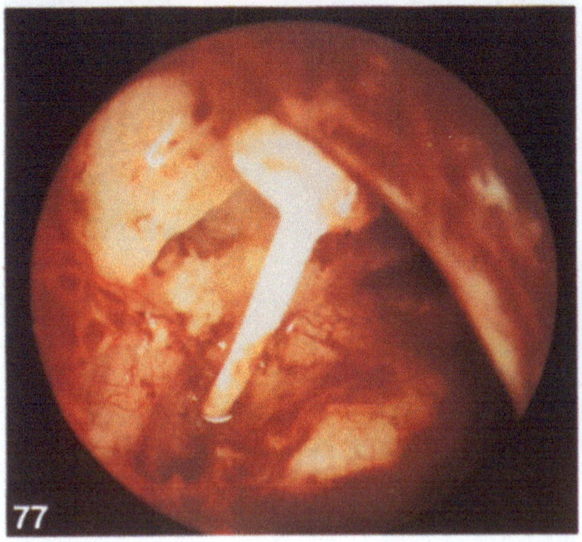

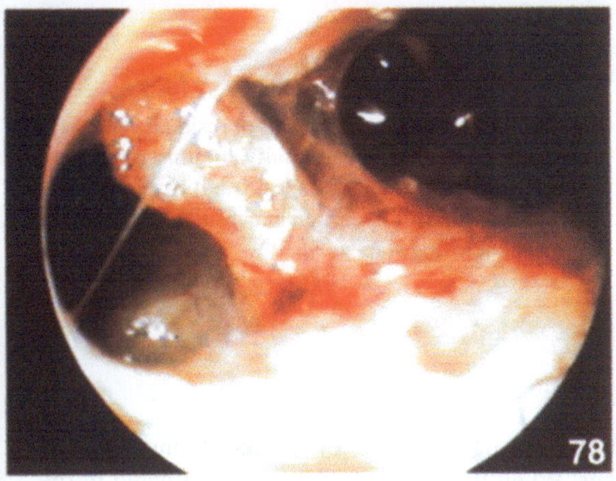

Fig. 76 a-d. Right ear: residual pearl in region of stapes (videoprint). **a** View of residual pearl through posterior tympanotomy window, 0° optical system; **c** view of tympanic cavity and pearl, 0° system; **d** monitoring after guided endoscopic excision of pearl

Fig. 77. Right ear: mallear prosthesis; 0° angle monitoring of position of stem of prosthesis in relation to base-plate

Fig. 78. Right ear: monitoring of ossiculoplasty with lens system passed through posterior tympanotomy (videoprint)

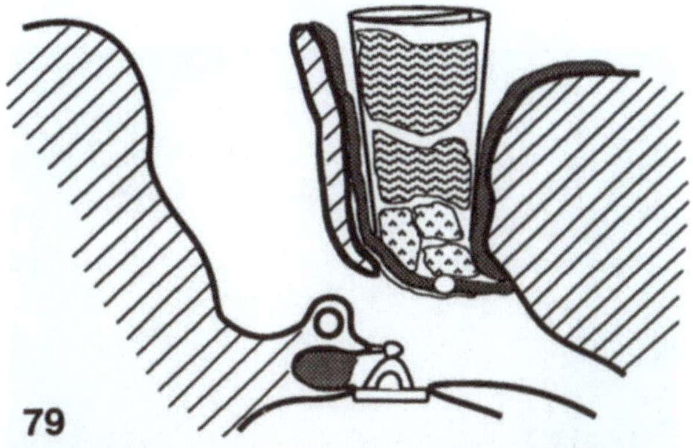

79

Fig. 79. Dressing of EAM. Rolled silastic with gelfoam

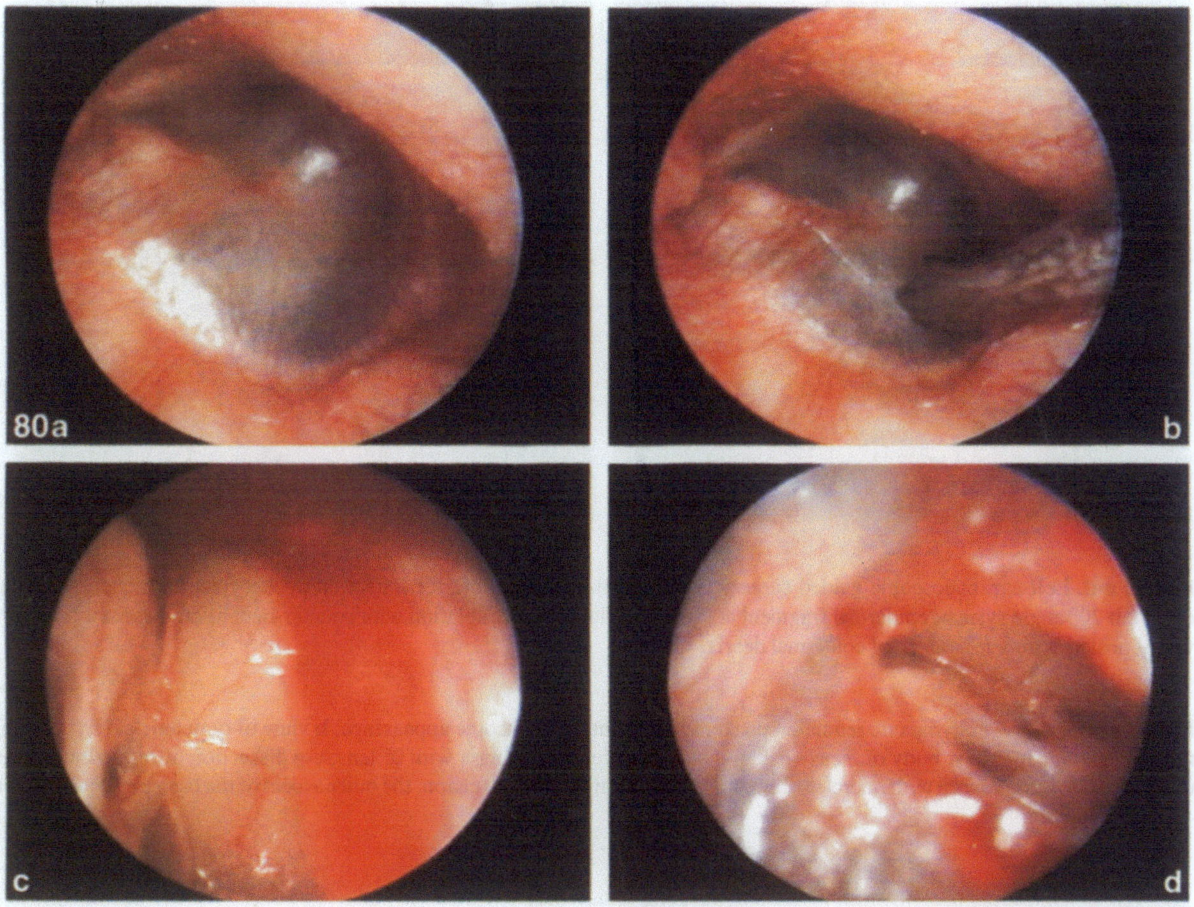

Fig. 80 a-d. Right ear: second stage monitoring of tympanic cavity via myringotomy (videoprint). **a, b** 0° system: myringotomy in posteroinferior quadrant; **c** 0° system: visualisation of incudo-stapedial region; **d** 70° system: inspection of retrotympanum

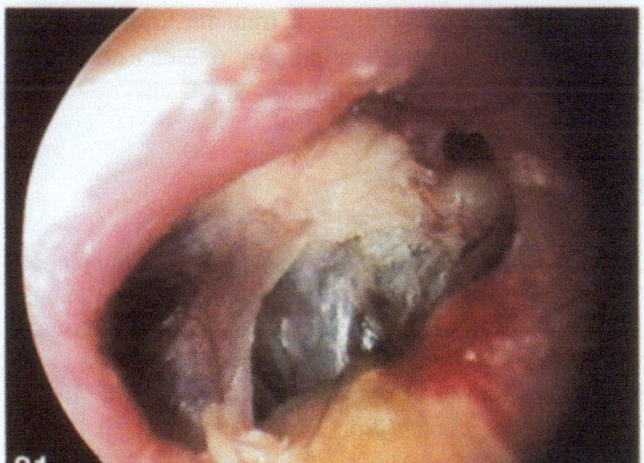

Fig. 81. Left ear: posterior retraction pocket (videoprint)

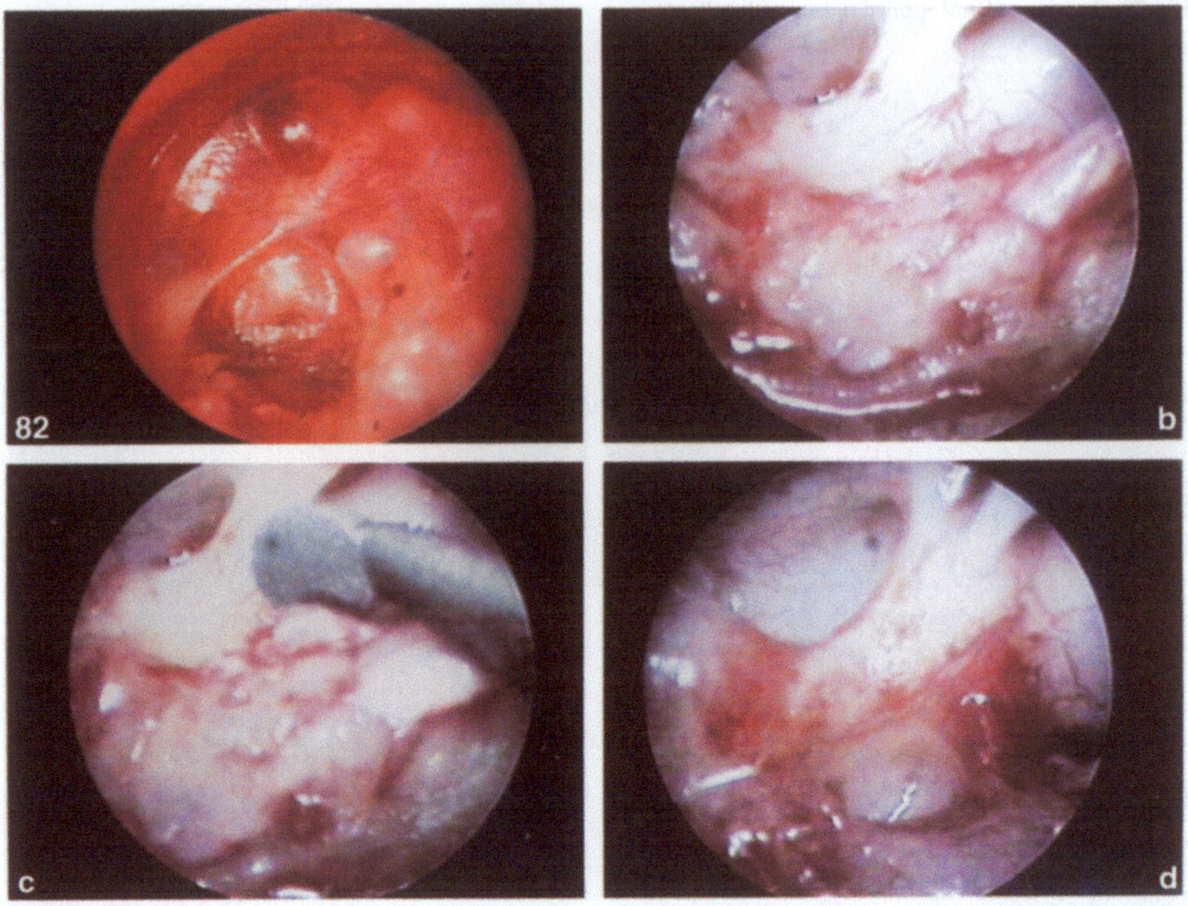

Fig. 82 a-d. Left ear: endoscopic guided surgery (videoprint). **a** Posteroinferior retraction pocket fixed to incudo-stapedial region; **b** 70° angle system: epidermal fragment at level of facial recess; **c** ablation with counter-bent microdissector final survey of posterior gutter: absence of epidermal debris

→

Fig. 83 a-h. Left ear: epitympanic retraction pocket (videoprint). **a** Otoscopic appearance; **b** view of tympanic cavity; **c** spontaneous epitympanotomy: body of incus visible; **d** survey of retrotympanum with 0° lens; **e-g** dissection of retraction pocket under endoscopic guidance with micro-instrument; h inspection at end of excision: the outer aspect of the ossicular mass is seen

block, we prefer to choose a transmastoid surgical approach, since with an atticotomy one can never be sure of reaching the base of the pocket.

References

Dubreuil C, Boulud B, Dumourest D (1991) Intérêt de l'otoendoscopie dans le traitement des deuxièmes temps de cholestéatome de l'oreille moyenne. Rev Laryngol Otol Rhinol (Bord) 112 : 409-411

Freche Ch, Rouvier P, Piquet JJ, Thomassin JM (1989) Endoscopie diagnostique et thérapeutique en ORL. Rapport à la Société Française d'ORL de Pathologie Cervico-faciale. Arnette, Paris pp 339-402

Horn K, Brackmann D, Luxford W, Shea J (1986) The supratubal recess in cholesteatoma surgery. Ann Otol Rhinol Laryngol 95 : 12-15

Mc Kennan K (1993) Endoscopic second look mastoidoscopy to rule out residual epitympanic mastoid cholesteatoma. Laryngoscope 103 : 810-814

Marquet J (1989) My current cholesteatoma techniques. Am J Otol 10 : 124-130

Martin Ch, Prades JM, Mayaud R, Calloch F (1993) Endoscopie et chirurgie des poches de rétraction tympaniques. J Fr ORL 42 : 315-319

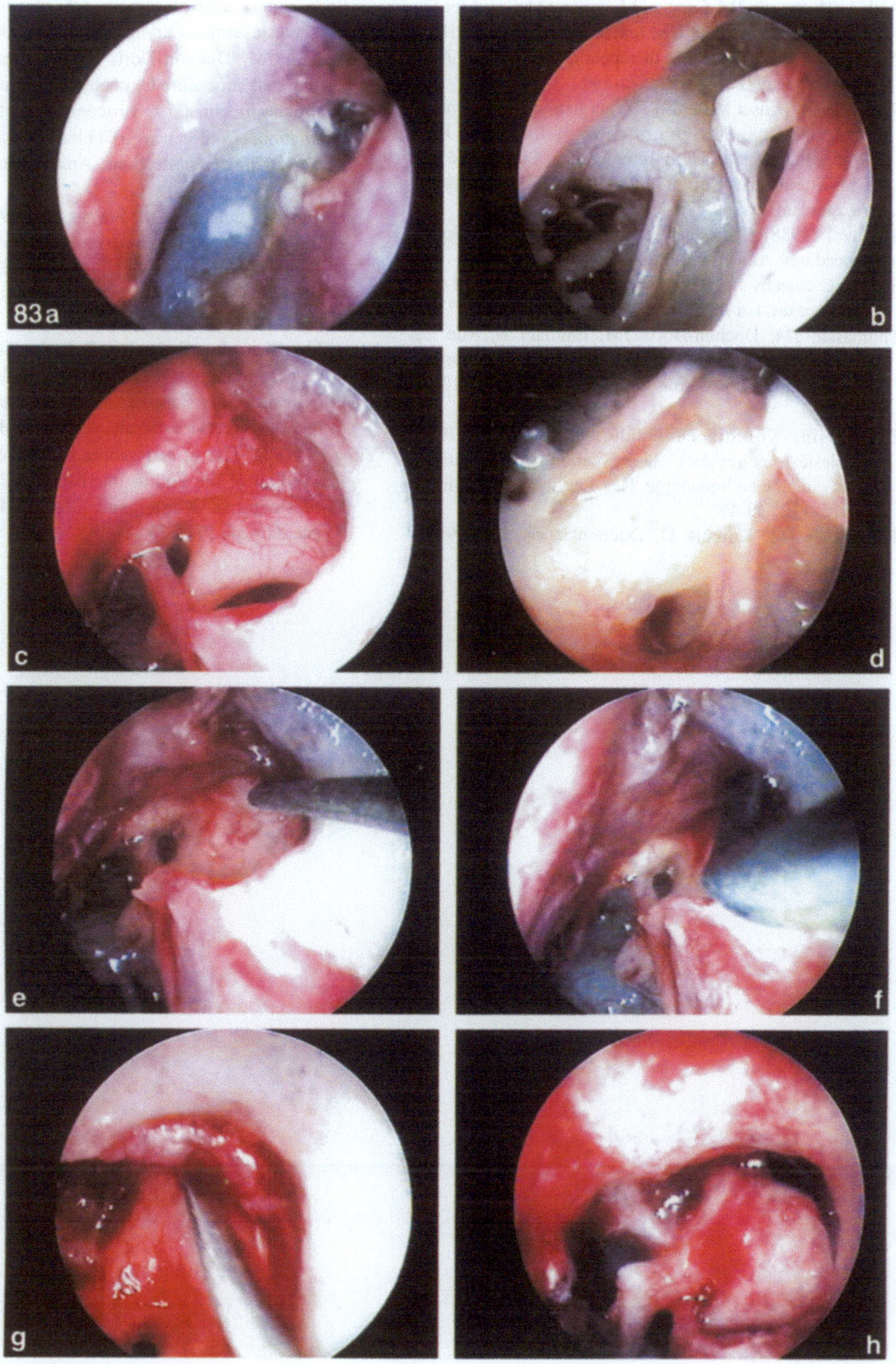
83a
b
c
d
e
f
g
h

Pech A, Thomassin JM, Cannoni M, Zanaret M, Scavenec C, Triglia JM (1985) Cholestéatome de l'oreille. Expérience d'une attitude thérapeutique éclectique. Ann Otol Laryngol (Paris) 102 : 575-580

Schinotler R, Lanser M (1989) The surgical management of cholesteatoma. The contribution of the laser. In : Proceeding of the Third International Conference on Cholesteatoma. Kugler and Ghedini Publications, Amsterdam, pp 769-778

Sheehy J (1988) Cholesteatoma surgery canal wall down procedures. Ann Otol Rhinol Laryngol 97 : 30-35

Shelton C, Sheehy J (1990) Tympanoplasty : review of 400 staged cases. Laryngoscope 100 : 679-681

Thomassin JM, Duchon-Doris JM, Emmam B, Ruc C, Conciatori J, Vilcoq P (1990) Otochirurgie endoscopique premier bilan. Ann Otol Laryngol (Paris) 107 : 564-570

Thomassin, Korchia D, Duchon-Doris JM (1991) Cholestéatome résiduel : sa prévention par la chirurgie sous guidage endoscopique. Rev Laryngol Otol Rhinol (Bord) 112 : 43-45

Thomassin JM, Korchia D, Duchon-Doris JM (1993) Endoscopic guided otosurgery in the prevention of residual cholesteatomas. Laryngoscope 103 : 939-943

Thomassin JM, Duchon-Doris JM, Korchia D (1993) Second look procedure for cholesteatoma using otovideoendoscopic surgery. Proceedings of the fourth International Conference on Cholesteatoma and Mastoïd Surgery. Kugler Publications, Amsterdam, New York, pp 502-506

Vandeventer G, Juantegui M, Fraysse B (1991) Interest of endoscopy in cholesteatoma revision. Politzer Society Conference on the Reality in Ear Surgery and Otoneurosurgery, Maastricht, Netherlands, june 16-21, 1991

Wayoff M, Charachon R, Rouleau P, Lacher G, Deguine Ch (1982) Le traitement chirurgical du cholesteatome de l'oreille moyenne. Rapport à la Société Française d'ORL de Pathologie cervico-faciale, Arnette, Paris

Yung M (1992) Use of endoscopes in middle ear surgery. Proceeding of the Fourth International Conference on Cholesteatoma. Kugler and Ghedini Publications, Amsterdam, pp 577-579

Indications

Surgery of cholesteatoma

Classic otologic surgery under operative microscopy has proved to have its limitations, whatever the technique. It is performed blindly and thus adds to the risk of residual cholesteatoma. It is especially in this form of otitic pathology that use of the endoscope is properly indicated, and with two objectives:

– monitoring of the quality of eradication;

– supplementing the operating microscope surgery with a video-monitored procedure.

In closed-technique tympanoplasties (the "canal wall up" procedure)

Here, the approach to the cholesteatoma is by a transmastoid route which respects the intactness of the EAM. (This technique implies the creation of a posterior tympanotomy window).

During the first operative stage

In modern otologic surgery one must have available endoscopic monitoring of the mastoid and tympanic cavities with optical systems of 0°, 30° and 70° angle and 2.7 mm diameter, and this whatever the experience of the operator (fig. 84 a-c). Since 1988 we have performed 55 first stage procedures for cholesteatoma by closed technique. In 40 cases endoscopic monitoring showed that excision of the epidermal mucosa under the microscope had been satisfactory, a result confirmed by endoscopy. On the other hand, in 15 cases (28%) we have had to supplement the procedure by otovideoendoscopic surgery.

Thus, the use of an optical system has proved essential in nearly one case in three. This was the case in the anterior epitympanum as well as in the retrotympanum. Hence, the contribution of otovideoendoscopy is that of a technique supplementary to the operating microscope in obtaining an "ideal" excision. It reduces the risk percentage for residual cholesteatoma during conservative tympanoplasty of the bony auditory channel.

During the second operative stage

During the second operative stage of a closed-technique tympanoplasty for cholesteatoma endoscopy can either:

– monitor the "blind" zones during a classical stage by the posterior route under operative microscopy or

– allow a minimal retroauricular cutaneous approach.

CT examination by axial and coronal sections, requested a month before operation, has guided us in our choice of the cutaneous approach. If the scan appearances identifies free air-containing cavities or a partial opacity, monitoring is initiated by a minimal retroauricular cutaneous approach (cf. preceding chapter) (fig. 85 a, b). Should there be a major recurrence, we abandoned purely endoscopic surgery and enlarged the cutaneous approach, as in a classical route of approach, to resume use of the operating microscope. A limited recurrence in the form of a pearl may sometimes, depending on its position, be removed under endoscopic guidance by the minimal route of access.

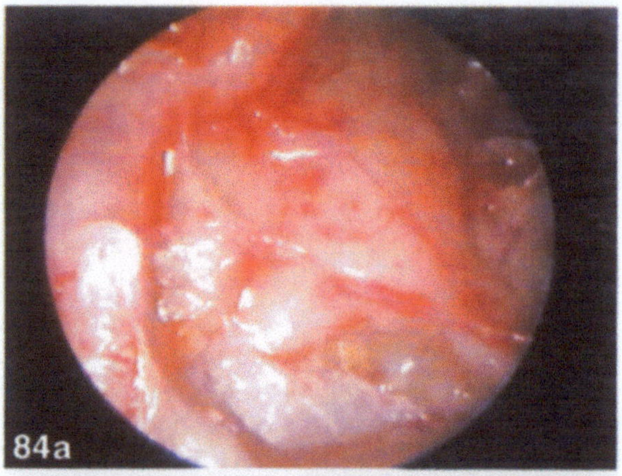

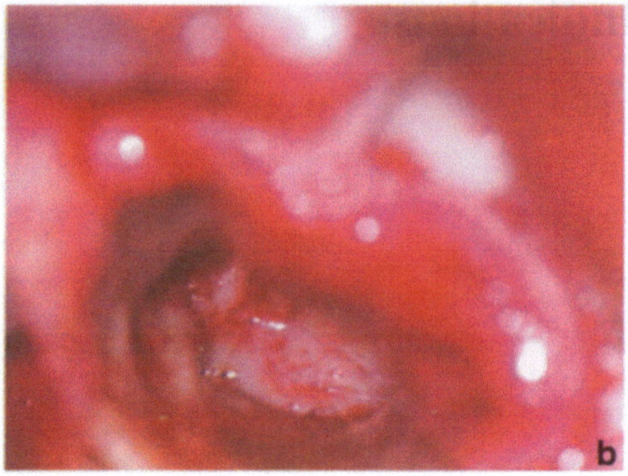

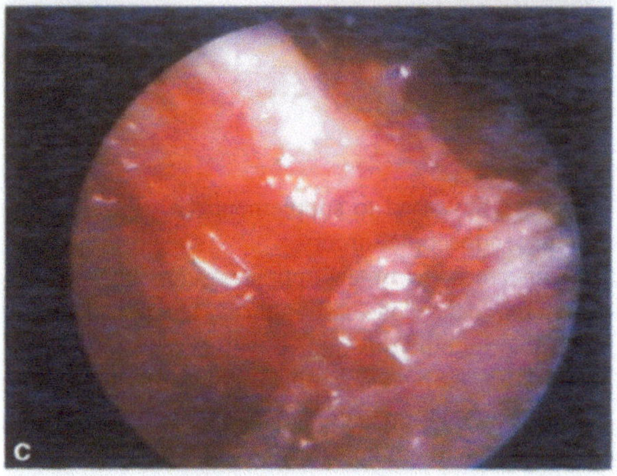

Fig. 84 a-c. Right ear: epidermosis of tympanic cavity (videoprint). **a** Survey with 0° system, epidermal debris present; **b** view with operating microscope (magnification x 16); **c** the 70° system demonstrates an epidermal plaque at the retrotympanum

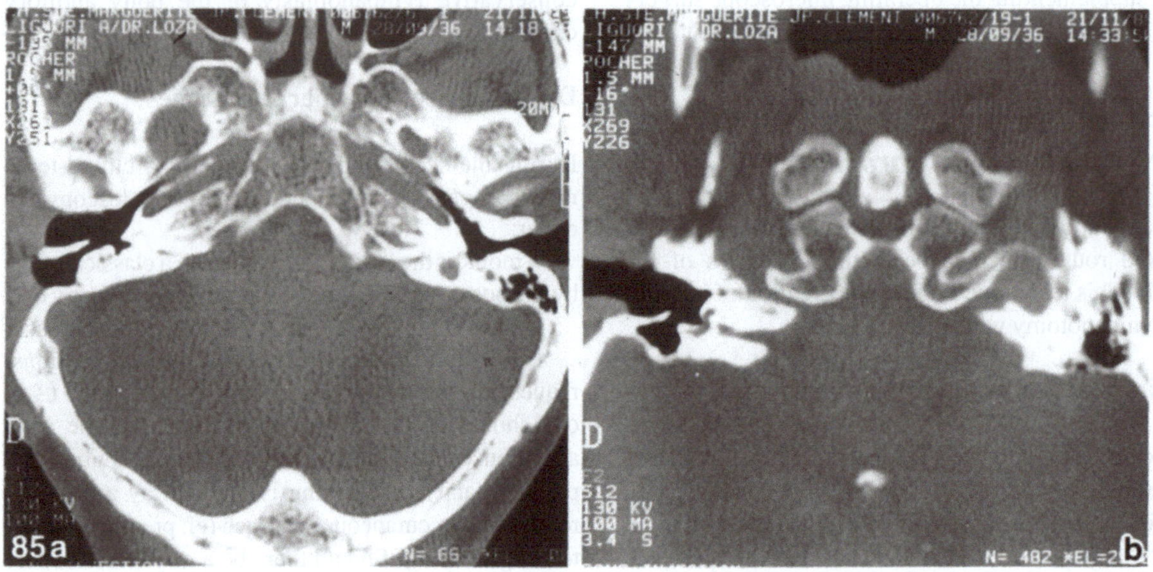

Fig. 85 a,b. Preoperative CT (one month before second stage surgery). **a** Horizontal section through posterior tympanotomy window: free air-filled cavity; **b** frontal section: absence of opacity at level of tympanic cavity

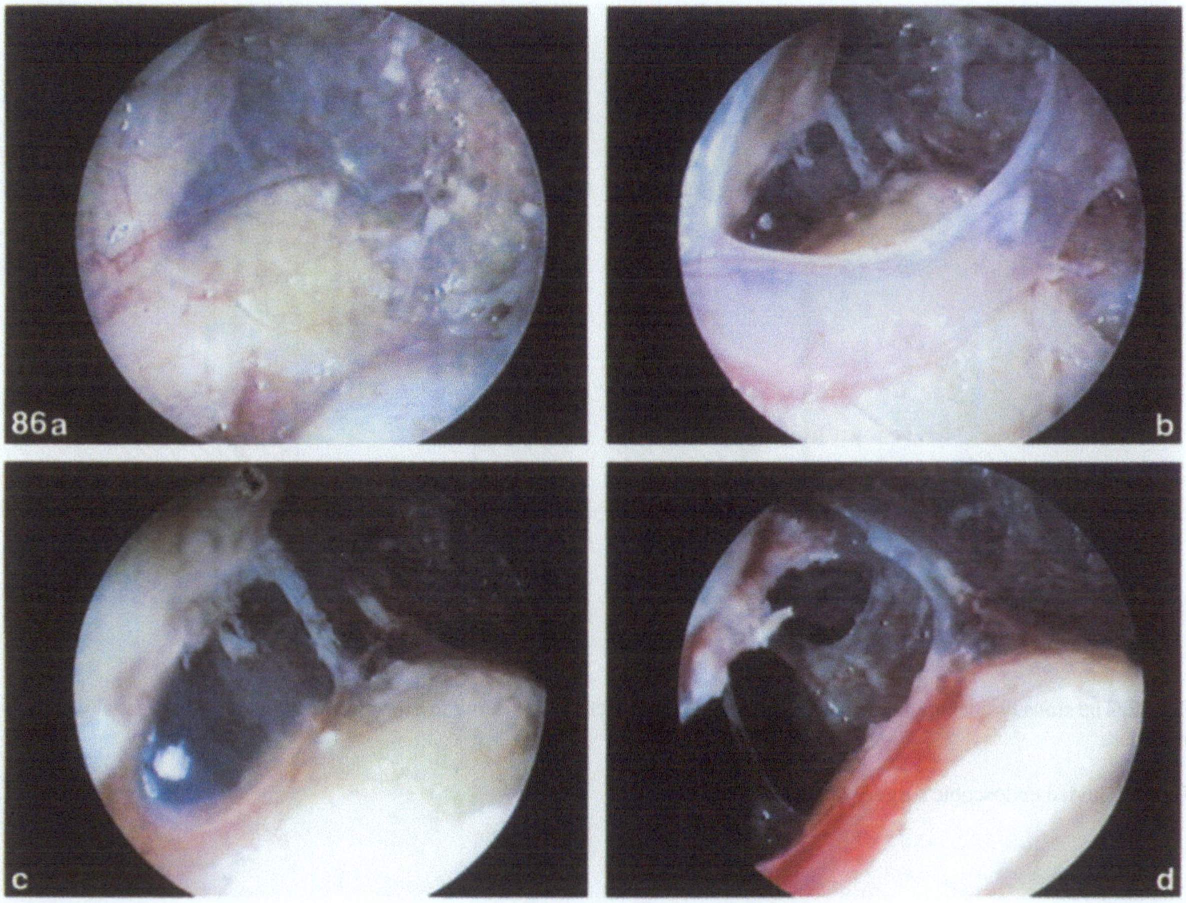

Fig. 86 a-d. Right ear: endoscopic monitoring of tympano-mastoid cavities at second stage of closed technique (videoprint). **a, b** Meshwork clothing mastoid cavity; **c** posterior tympanotomy window obstructed by fine veil; **d** after opening, the head of the stapes is seen

The advantages of such endoscopic surgical revision under video monitoring are many:

– first, this check can be made under day surgery conditions, with local or general anesthesia. The absence of postoperative dressings permits earlier professional revision, so that a second stage is more acceptable to the patients

– amatomically, video-monitored surgery also provides a great degree of security in the assessment of the mastoid and epitympanic cavities (fig. 86 a-d). This approach is atraumatic for the lining mucosa of the posterior cavities of the middle ear. This checking by a minimal retroauricular procedure is often combined with exploration via the EAM in order to monitor the tympanic cavity and, if necessary, allows an ossiculoplasty.

Since 1990 we have performed 35 revision operations using this technique without encountering any difficulty at opening the mastoid. However, should there be any ossification, it is very simple to use a burr to abrade the newly-formed bone.

In open-technique tympanoplasties (the "canal wall down" procedure)

Removal of the posterior wall of the bony auditory canal only very slightly improves the view of the posterior sulcus of the tympanic cavity. When the sinus tympani is deep, it remains inaccessible to view under the operating microscope (fig. 87). Monitoring of the depths of the cavity, in cases of epidermosis or cholesteatoma extend-

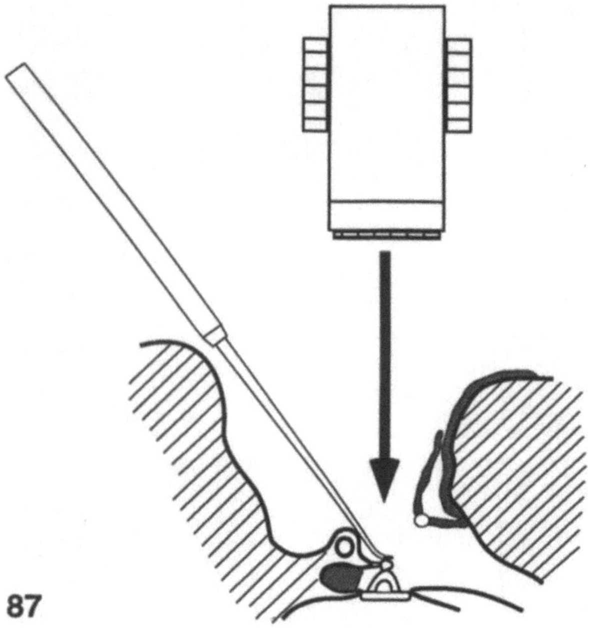

87

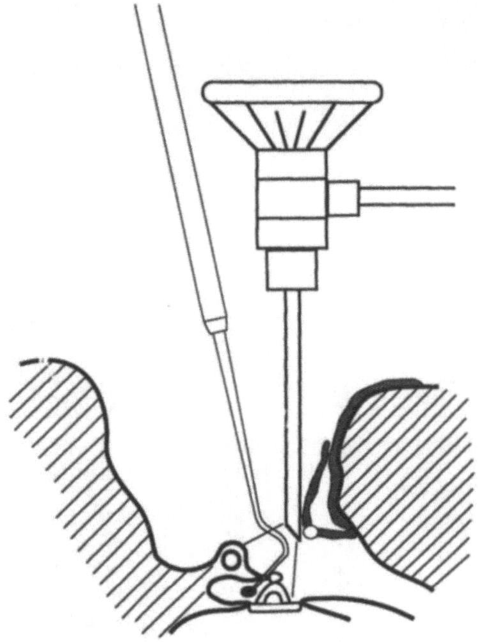

88

Fig. 87. The sinus tympani remains inaccessible to vision under the operating microscope even in the case of canal wall down procedure

Fig. 88. Guided endoscopic surgery of sinus tympani

ing to this region, is impossible. This is particularly common in certain cholesteatomas in children.

Therefore, in every case where the so-called "open" technique is used, we advise routine checking of this region with 30° and 70° optical systems (fig. 88).

Epidermatisation of the tympanic cavity

The epidermis may glide insidiously, starting from the margin of the perforation (fig. 89 a-c), to spread over the long process and the head of the stapes. Sometimes the handle of the malleus, at the center of a perforation, is prolonged by an epidermal sheet (fig. 90 a-h) which ascends along the inner aspect of the handle of the malleus towards its neck. These two sorts of cases provide the justification for peroperative endoscopic monitoring since this allows more certain excision of this epidermis, especially when this has a tendency to flow as a sheet towards the retrotympanum.

Retraction pockets

Posterior and posterior subligamentous invaginations constitute an excellent indication for guided endoscopic surgery. Their excision may then be effected by the transmeatal route without any need for a transmastoid posterior route.

The situation is quite different with the invaginations of Schrapnell and of the anterior subligamentous region. While excision of the pocket by way of the EAM is sometimes satisfactory, it is usually necessary to choose a transmastoid route with anterior tympanotomy, or else an epitympanotomy by the transmeatal route with preservation of a rod tailored from the bony margin, and reconstruction of the attic wall by a fragment of bone, cartilage or biomaterial.

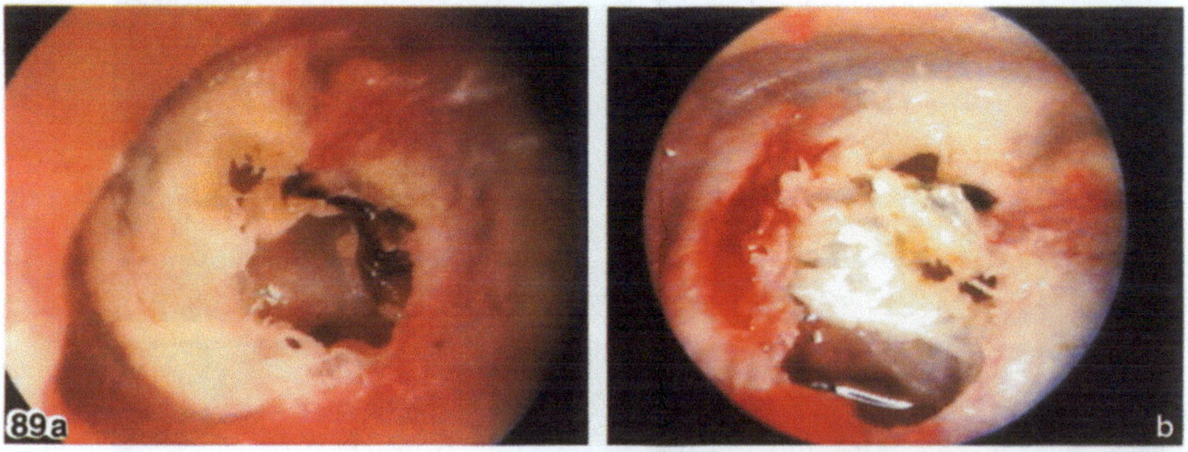

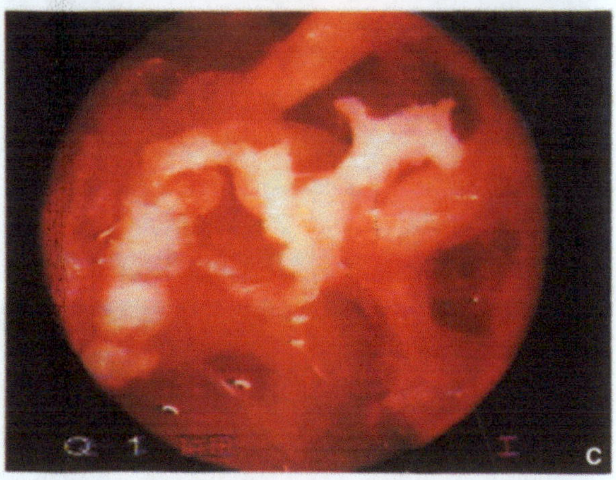

Fig. 89 a-c. Left ear: mediotympanic epidermosis (videoprint). **a** Cholesteatoma developing from a tympanic perforation; **b** otoscopic view through perforation with 0° optical system. Note presence of epidermal flow in incudo-stapedial region; **c** peroperative view of layered epidermal involvement of incudo-stapedial region

Techniques for reconstruction of old radical cavity

We have considered it legitimate to use the endoscopic equipment to monitor ablation of the epidermis at the retro- and protympanum. Sometimes, the origin of the indications for these techniques is an otorrhea, which may indicate either the recurrence of a cholesteatoma or defective epidermisation of the cavity, or else the presence of an epidermis clothing the protympanic region. In old radical cavity, it is absolutely necessary before any bony reconstruction to ensure complete epidermal excision in the tympanic cavity. Here, too, the use of peroperative endoscopy is indicated (fig. 91 a, b).

Ossiculoplasties

When the columellar restoration is completed, peroperative use of endoscopy seems useful for confirming perfect placement of the prosthetic system (fig. 92), more particularly in ossiculoplasties of Wullstein's type III, where one can verify proper positioning of the prosthesis on the footplate of the stapes by use of a system of 0° angle and 2.7 mm diameter.

After having reflected the tympanomeatal flap and completed the dressing via the meatus in transmastoid surgery, we take the precaution, by means of 30° and 70° angle optical systems, to verify the absence of slipping of the ossicular set-up and also its position in relation to the bony margin, the handle of the malleus or, if these are absent, to the tympanic membrane.

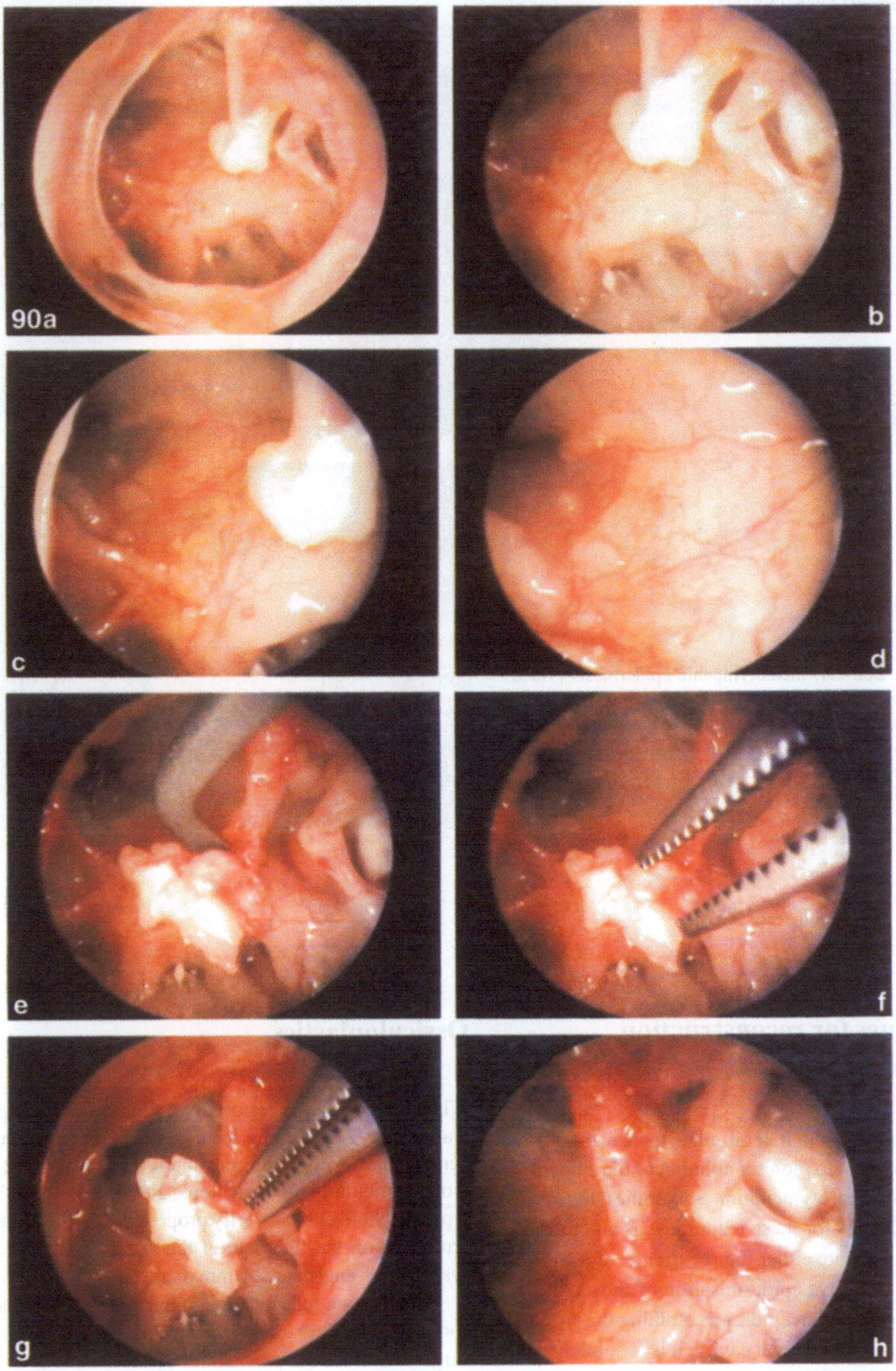

Fig. 90 a-h, Left ear: epidermosis situated at handle of malleus (videoprint). **a-c** Subtotal marginal perforation related to handle of malleus with epidermal debris; **d** survey of protympanum; **e-g** dissection of cholesteatomatous matrix from handle of malleus under endoscopic guidance; **h** monitoring of eradication with 30° lens system in the region of the cochleariform process

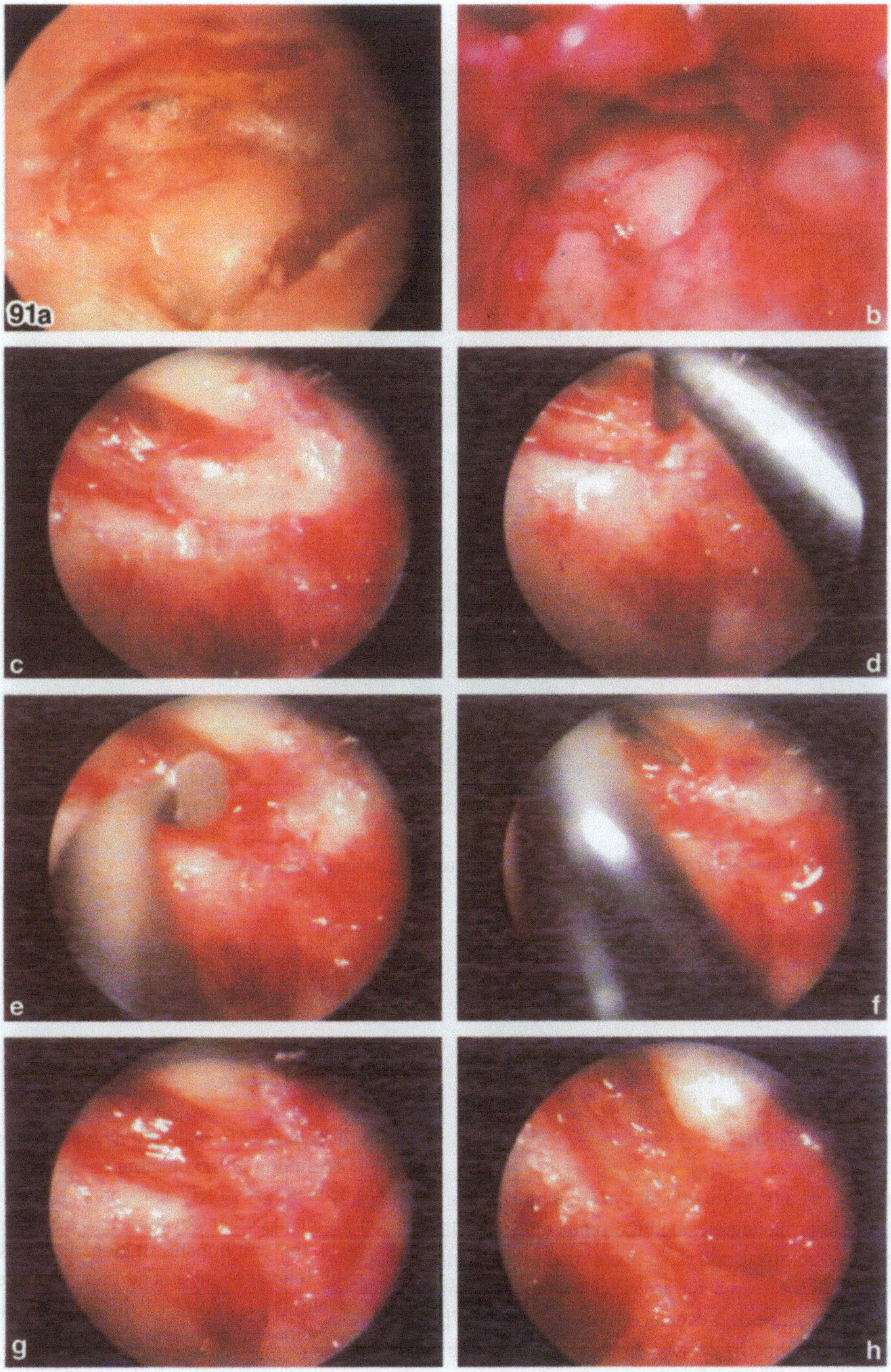

Fig. 91 a-h. Right ear: reconstruction of old radical cavity (videoprint). **a** Epidermis molding medial wall of tympanic cavity; **b** view of tympanic cavity with operating microscope after ablation of epidermis; **c, d** the 70° lens system demonstrates a residual epidermal fragment at the retrotympanum; **e-g** dissection of epidermal residue using optical system; **h** monitoring of region of sinus tympani at end of operation: note absence of epidermal debris

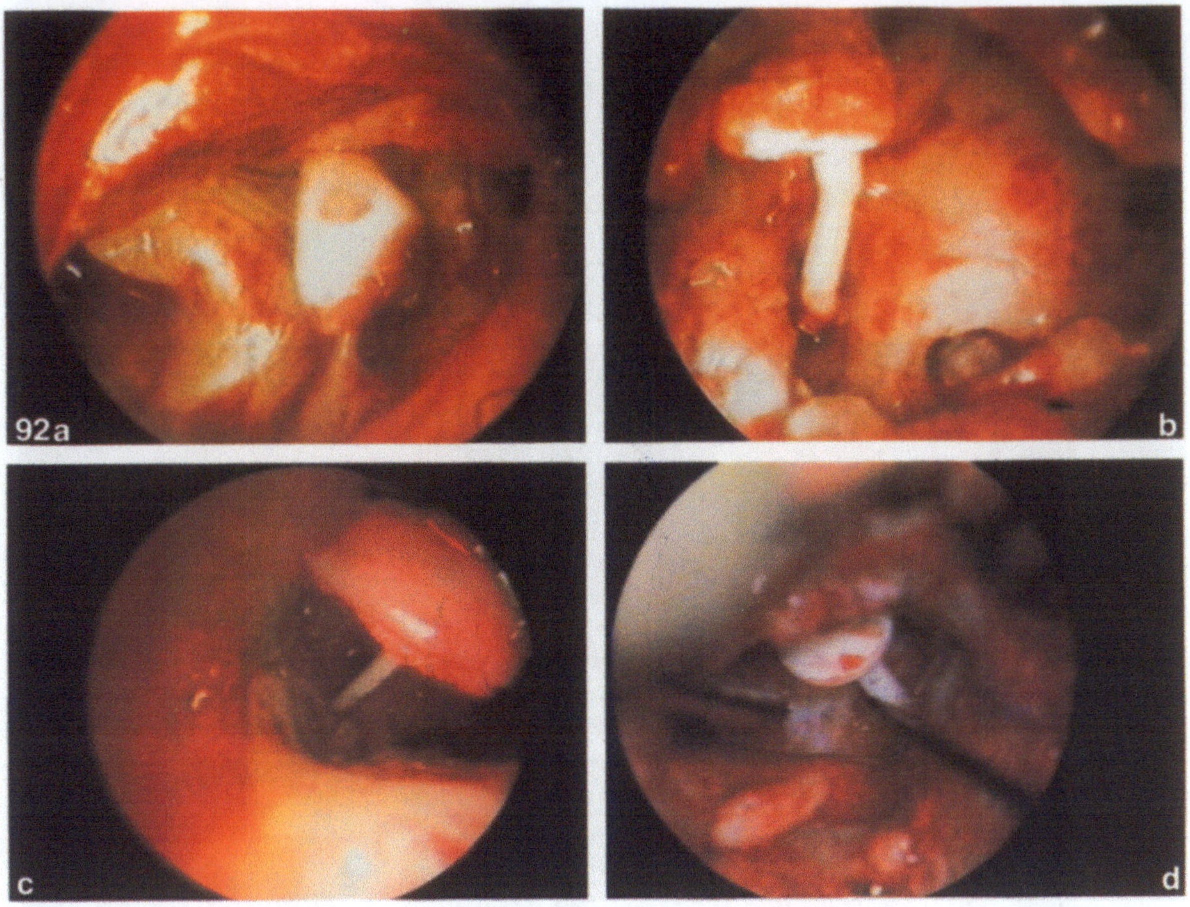

Fig. 92. Monitoring under 0° optical system of different ossicular arrangements (videoprint)

Congenital malformations

Minor aplasias

Insertion of a 0° angle optical system in the tympanic cavity, after having elevated the tympanomeatal flap, permits a complete and rapid inventory of the existing ossicles in the search for an ossicular anomaly (malleus, incus, stapes), or even agenesis (fig. 93 a-d). This exploration exactly defines the course of the facial nerve and verifies the functioning of the incudo-stapedial joint, without there being any need to damage the bony frame of the EAM. The observation of a reflection at the round window, under the lens, confirms the functional character of the ossicular chain.

Major aplasias

The technique of creating a new bony auditory channel, beginning at the opening of the mastoid cavities, has been progressively abandoned. Like other authors, we prefer to center our burring by following the tegmen of the epitympanic region. Progressive careful burring related to the linea temporalis opens the epitympanic cavity, where a malformed fused incudo-mallear bloc is often found.

The use of an oblique optical system in the trench thus created allows a rapid definition of the position of the facial nerve, the existence or not of an incudo-stapedial joint and the presence of a stapedial superstructure (fig. 94 a-d), The enlargement of the new channel is then carried out from above downwards, and from

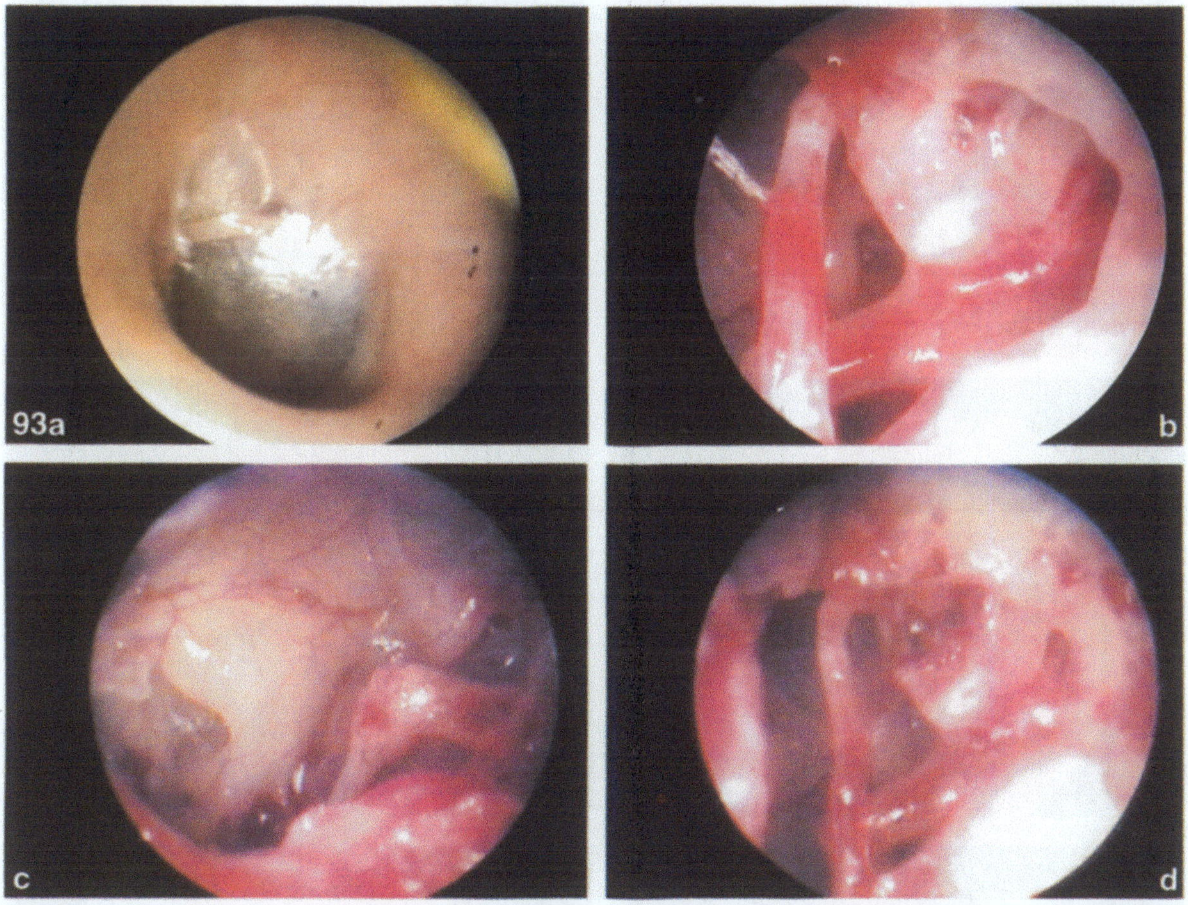

Fig. 93 a-d. Left ear: minor aplasia (videoprint). **a** Otoscopic appearance: absence of handle of malleus; **b** mallear bloc fixed to anterior wall of EAM; **c** survey of incudo-stapedial joint under 30° optical system; **d** final appearance after section of bony bridge tethering region of neck of malleus to wall of EAM

behind forward, with the burr and is completed by ablation of the atresic plaque with the microcurette.

Other applications

Search for a perilymphatic fistula

Surgical exploration of the window region takes place by a transmeatal route under local or general anesthesia. These fistulas are often difficult to locate under operative microscopy. The luminosity and wide visual field of the optical systems make them a valuable aid for the surgeon treating deafness Indeed, the use of these optical systems allows demonstration of the fluid that wells up outside the perilymphatic fistula.

They are usually localised in the region of the (oval) window. Using the system of 0° angle, special attention is given to the zone of the antefenestral fistula, which is situated at the anterior pole of the oval window. They may also exist at the (round) window. This is hollowed at the base of a fossula, the vanishing view of which under the operating microscope only rarely permits one to perceive the secondary tympanum. Using optical systems of 0° and 30° one can gain a view of the whole of the membrane sealing the round window (fig. 95 b, c), thus avoiding having to burr the ridge of the round window as frequently has to be done when using the operating microscope.

Thus, the availability of optical systems increases the chances of detecting such an anomaly, whether of congenital or, more usually, of traumatic origin.

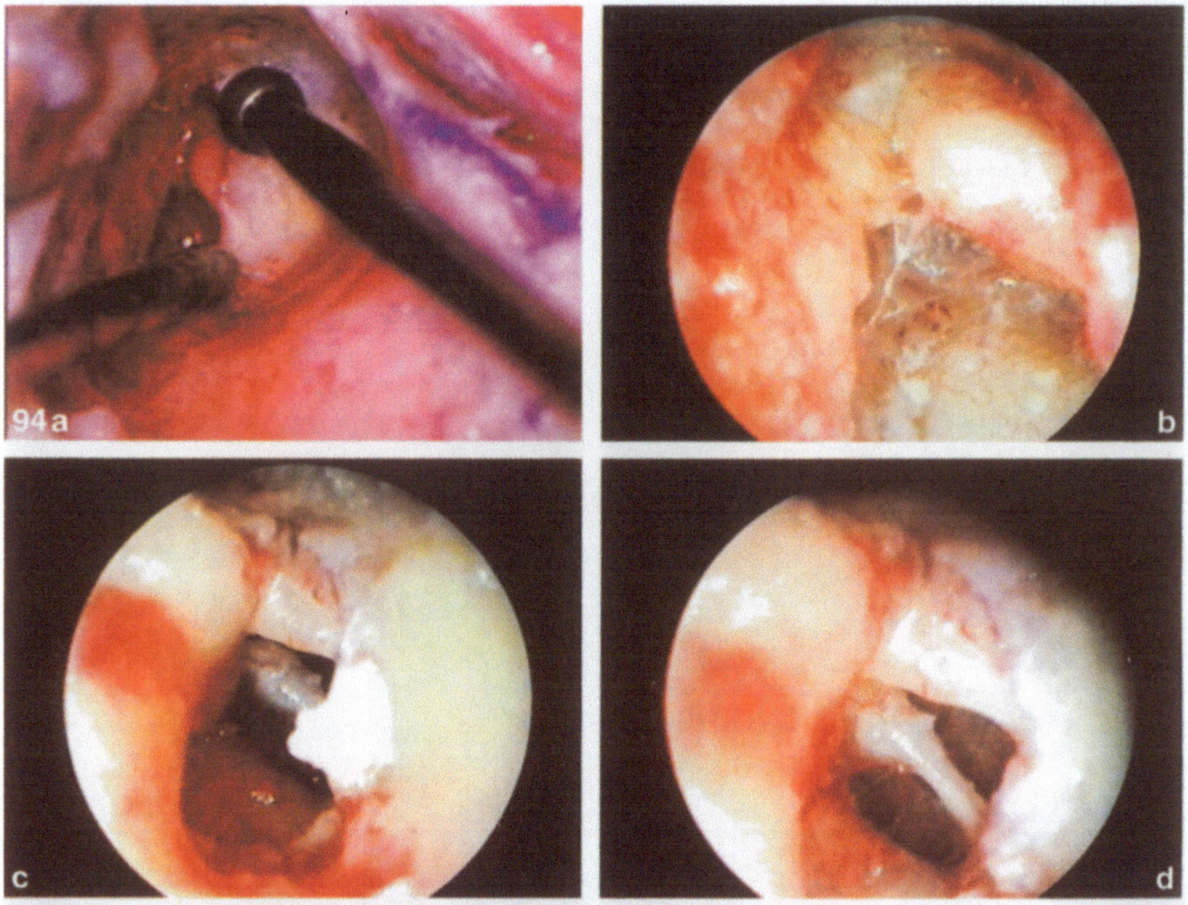
94 a
b
c
d

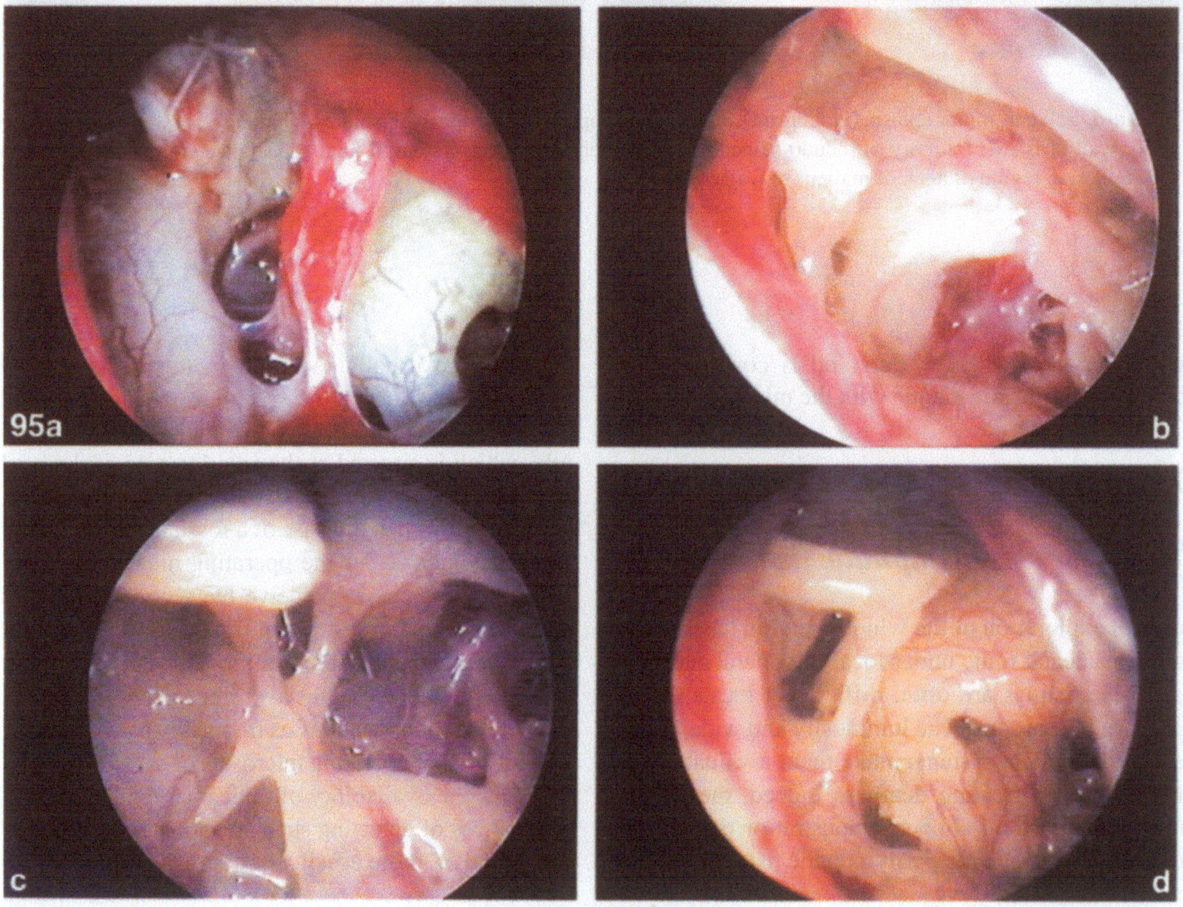
95a
b
c
d

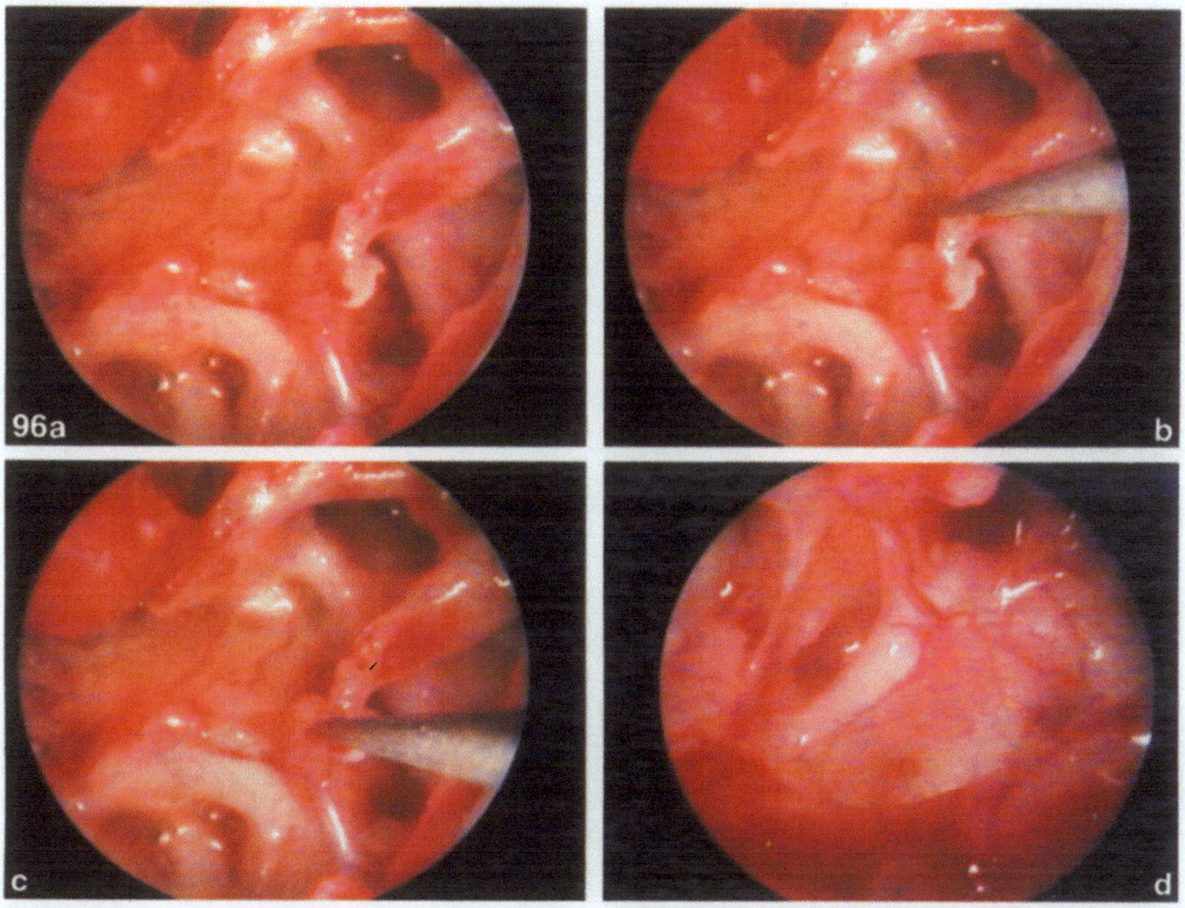

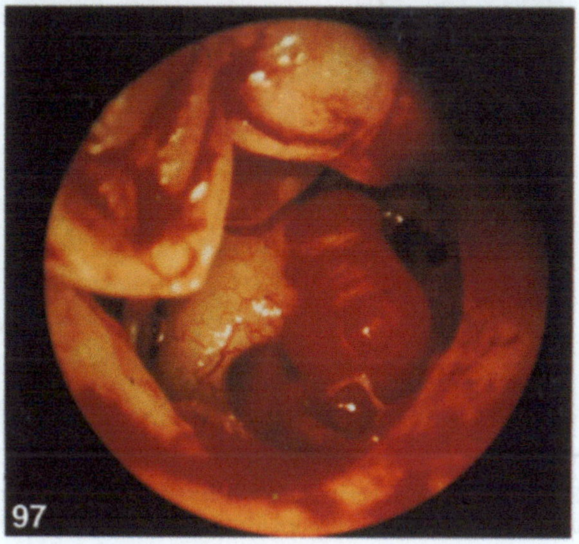

Fig. 96 a-d. Left ear: rupture of ossicular chain, incudo-stapedial disjunction (videoprint). **a-c** Incudo-stapedial disjunction, 0° optical systems; **d** search for reflection at secondary tympanum

Fig. 97. Right ear: tympanic paraganglioma

←

Fig. 94 a-d. Right ear: major aplasia (videoprint). **a** Burring of new channel centered on epitympanic region, operating microscope view; **b** identification of incudo-mallear joint, 0° optical system (image comparable with that of operating microscope); **c, d** view with 70° system before removal of atresic plaque; position of facial nerve and stapes visible

Fig. 95 a-d. Right ear: exploration of tympanic cavity in search for perilymphatic fistula (videoprint). **a** View of region of oval window. **b-d** different appearances of cochlear niche; **c** view of round window, 70° optical system

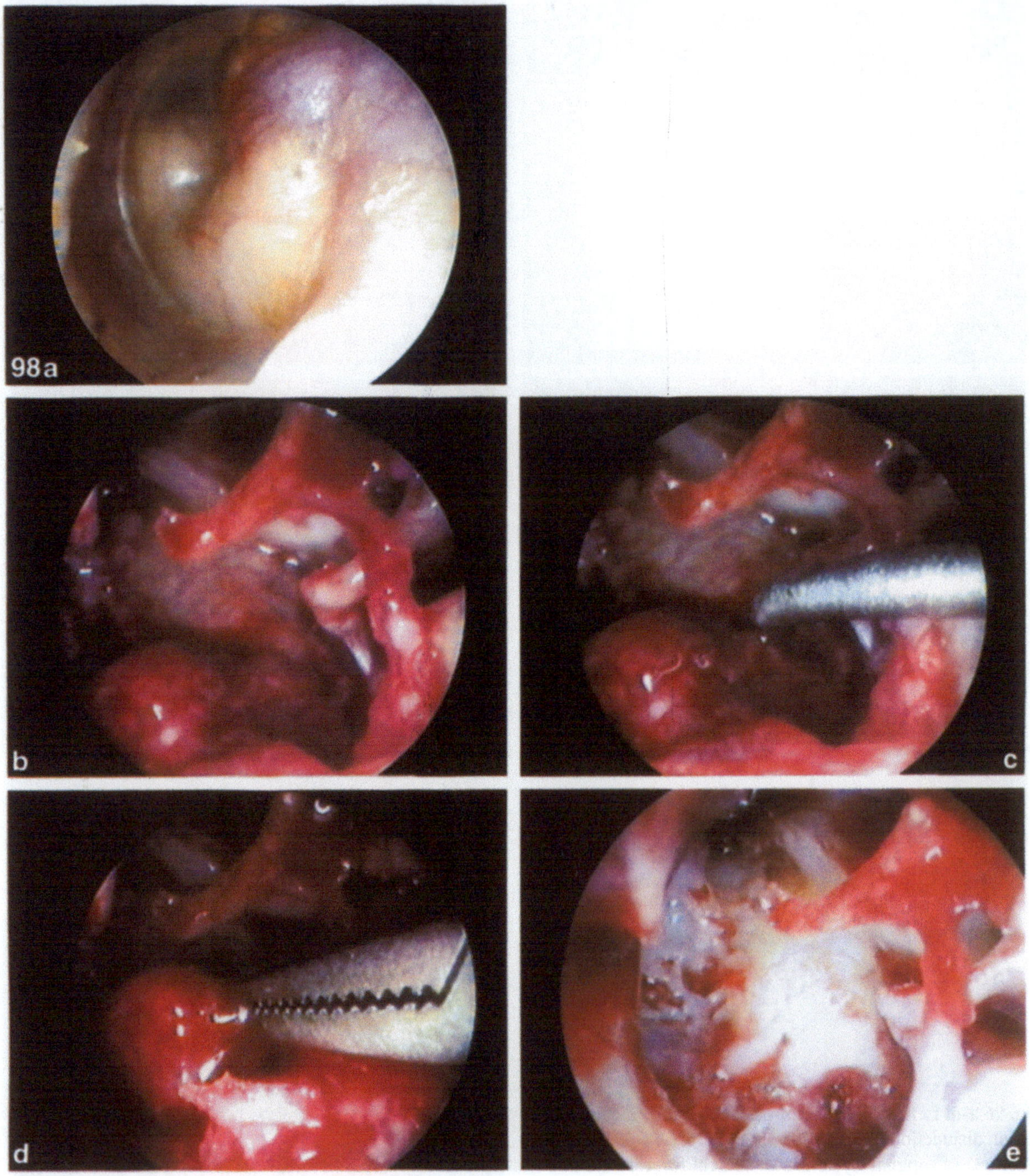

Fig. 98 a-e. Left ear: benign tumor of ear (videoprint). **a** Tumor (benign adenoma) elevating tympanum in posterior region; **b-d** excision of tumor embedded in retrotympanum; **e** monitoring of cavity with 0° optical system at end of eradication

Injuries of the ossicular chain

Examination of the incudo-stapedial region is more precise with an optical system (fig. 96 a-d).

Surgery of benign tumors

The use of optical systems may also sometimes be justified in monitoring the quality of excision at the end of operation. We have used them in three cases of tympanic para-gangliomas (fig. 97), one of which thrust a prolongation towards the protympanum and invaded the entire sinus tympani. In another case there was a benign adenoma of the middle ear (fig. 98 a-e).

Altogether, there are numerous applications in the surgery of the middle ear. The routine use of optical systems at all tympanoplasties familiarises the surgeon with the endoscopic anatomy and provides a training for him to refine his manipulations for any type of endoscopic guided surgery using a 70° optical system. In the near future advances in manufacture will provide us with semi-rigid fibers, truly malleable optical systems that can be bent and will aid us to explore the remotest corners of the tympano-mastoid cavities more easily.

Results of endoscopic guided surgery in tympanoplasty for cholesteatoma

Case material

Between 1979 and 1991, 166 cases of cholesteatoma were operated by a single surgeon, This was therefore a uniform series. 125 cases had a closed-technique eradication. 41 cases underwent open-technique tympanoplasty, and 25% of these had a modified radical-cavity (fig. 99).

All of these 125 cases operated by a technique preserving the bony canal wall, 80 cases so far have had a second stage for monitoring after an interval of between 10 and 24 months from the first stage. During this period 14% were lost to follow-up and therefore were not subjected to this second stage procedure.

Since May of 1985 we have used 0° and 70° otoendoscopes for monitoring zones difficult of access with the operating microscope. Since 1988, endoscopic guided surgery with video monitoring has been developed during the first and second operative stages as a supplement to conventional surgery. From 1990, in some cases, we have begun to carry out the second stage under video monitoring, by minimal access routes under local or general anesthesia, and with a shortened stay in hospital.

Thus, our statistics relate to two periods, the first from 1979 to April 1985, the other from May 1985 to December 1991.

Distribution by age (table 1)

– First period (1979 to April 1985): 36 adults and 8 children underwent closed-technique tympanoplasty for cholesteatoma with monitoring at a second operative stage.

– Second period (May 1985 to December 1991): 24 adults and 12 children were operated by an identical technique.

Thus the total consists of 60 adults and 20 children aged 15 years or less. Normally, this latter population presents the more aggressive cholesteatomas, with a high risk of recurrence.

Macroscopic appearance and localisation (table 2)

The cholesteatoma presented in the form of a hernial sac or an epidermosis (15%). This latter gross appearance was always localised to the tympanic cavity. Unlike the cholesteatomatous sac it is unfortunately impossible to eradicate in block the entire matrix in the epidermatoses, which adds to the risk of residual pathology. In both series, the site of the cholesteatoma demonstrated a large number of flows in the retrotympanic region. In the first series, 19 antro-attical cholesteatomas were noted with flow in the tympanic cavity, as well as 6 epidermatoses of the cavity. In the second series, 14 cases had the same topography and the number of epidermatoses of the cavity was the same.

Results

Analysis of results by residual cholesteatomas (table 3)

Analysis of the residual cholesteatomas observed, whether in the form of a pearl or of a "candle-grease"

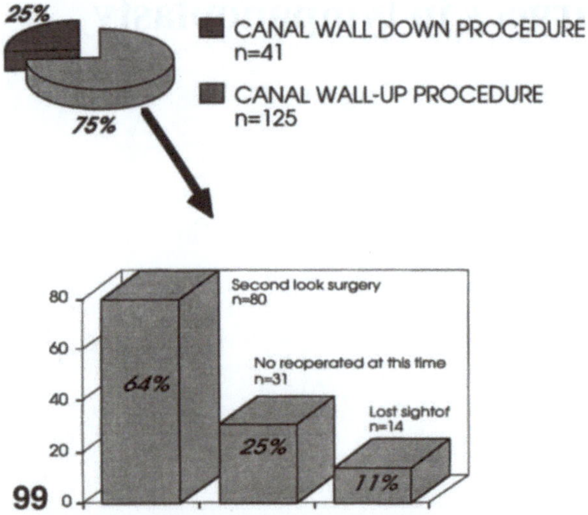

99

Fig. 99. The place of two-stage closed-technique tympanoplasty in tympanoplasties for cholesteatoma

Table 1. Cholesteatomas operated by closed-technique tympanoplasty in two stages (1979-1991: 80 cases)

	1979 – 1985 (4)	1985 (5) – 1991
Adults	36	24
Children	8	12
Total	44	36

Table 2. Localisation of cholesteatoma at closed-technique first stage operation

	1ère période 1979 – 1985 (4)	2ème période 1985 (5) – 1991
Cholesteatoma in hernial sac:		
Antrum + mastoid	13	9
Antrum + épitympanum + tympanum	19	14
Epitympanum	6	7
Epidermosis	6	6

epidermosis, yields a global figure of 47.7% without monitoring by endoscopic surgery as against 5.5% since the routine use of 0°, 30° and 70° optical systems. This significant variance in results, as between two comparable populations operated by the same surgeon, but with the eradication monitored by endoscopy in the second series, is a convincing argument for the progress achieved with this new technique. The precision brought by endoscopy is simply not to be compared with that given by stainless steel micro-mirrors.

On the other hand, the experience of the surgical

Table 3. Macroscopic appearances of residual cholesteatomas after closed technique in two stages 1979 – 1991: 80 cases

	1979 - 1985 (4) 44 cases unaided or micro-mirror		1985 (5) - 1991 36 cases otoendoscopy 0°, 70°	
Pearls	10	21/44 = 47,7 %	2	2/36 = 5,5 %
Epidermosis	11		0	

Table 4. Localisation of residual cholesteatomas

	1979 - 1985 (4) 21/44 cases		1985 (5) - 1991 2/36 cases	
	Pearl	Epidermosis	Pearl	Epidermosis
Appearance	10	11	2	0
Site:				
Mastoid	2	1	0	0
Epitympanum	4	3	0	0
Mesotympanum	4	7	2	0

otologist in 1979 already related to over 200 tympanoplasties, so that this is a factor which need not be taken into account in explaining the improvement in results.

The site of residual cholesteatomas

(table 4)

This is related to the topography of the initial cholesteatoma. We have stressed the difficulties we encountered in cleaning two regions: the anterior part of the epitympanum (supratubal fossula) and the retrotympanum. It is therefore not surprising that we found these two sites to be the preferential zones for the development of residual cholesteatoma in our first series. On the other hand, in the analysis of the second series, the two cases of residual cholesteatoma (both in the form of a pearl) appeared, one at the oval window and the other at the head of the stapes. However, we have not detected any recurrence at the region of the retrotympanum or of the epitympanum. In every case, guided endoscopic surgery has allowed us to perform a proper and more precise excision under visual monitoring in these difficultly accessed regions.

Frequency

In our series of cases monitored by peroperative endoscopy, no difference was observed between the numbers of encapsulated and epidermatotic forms of residual cholesteatomas. he development of a completely encapsulated pearl in the history of a patient with cholesteatoma is not serious. It is an event that can be foreseen and without serious consequences. These pearls have no destructive power, but, left in place for a long time, they simply become bulky and assume the appearance of a cholesteatomatous sac. With our strategy of routine revision this does not constitute a failure but only justifies our attitude.

On the other hand, in our first series 1 cases (25%) presented with an epidermosis, and 4 cases (9%) were sufficiently large to necessitate a third monitoring surgical stage. Nevertheless, during this period, we have never had to convert a closed technique into an open one.

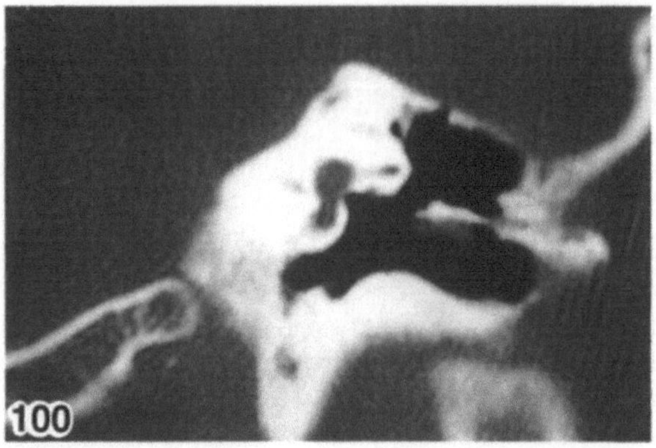

Fig. 100. High-resolution CT. Frontal section: perfectly free air-filled cavity

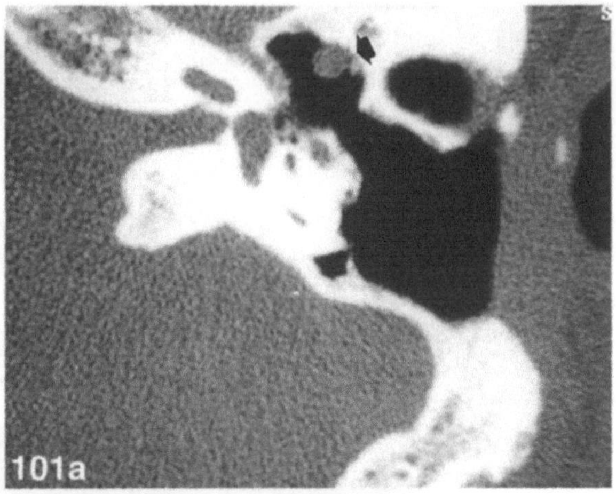

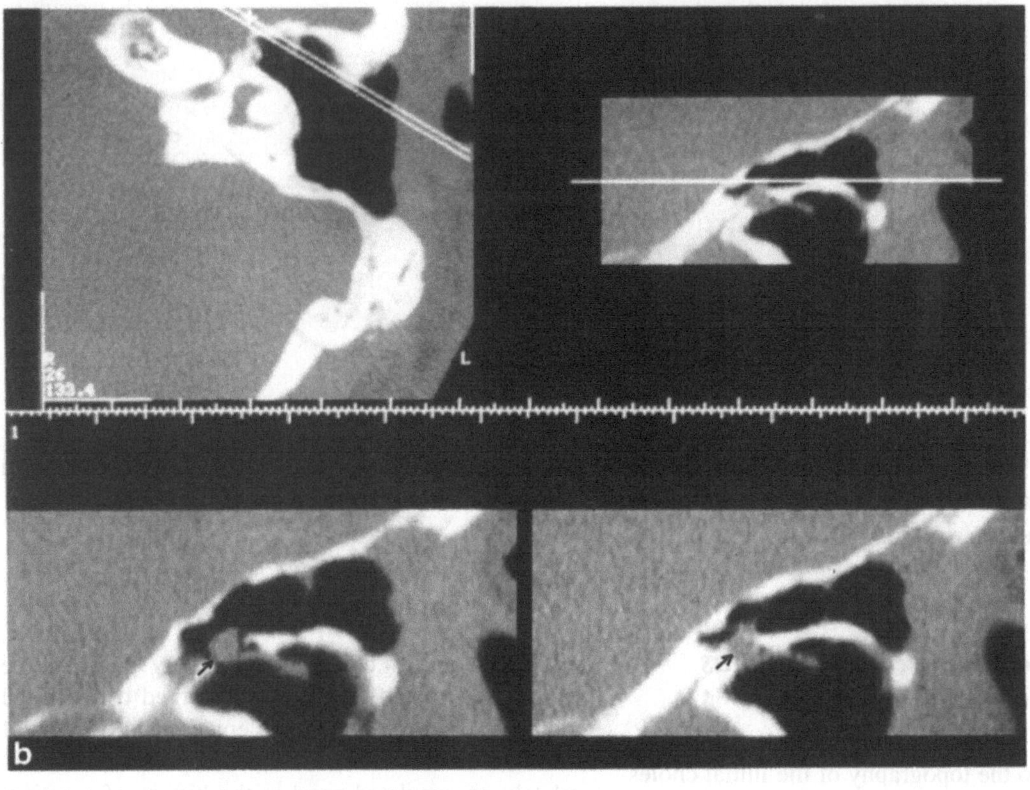

Fig. 101. High-resolution CT. Horizontal section: the arrow indicates a rounded isolated cavity, a residual pearl of cholesteatoma

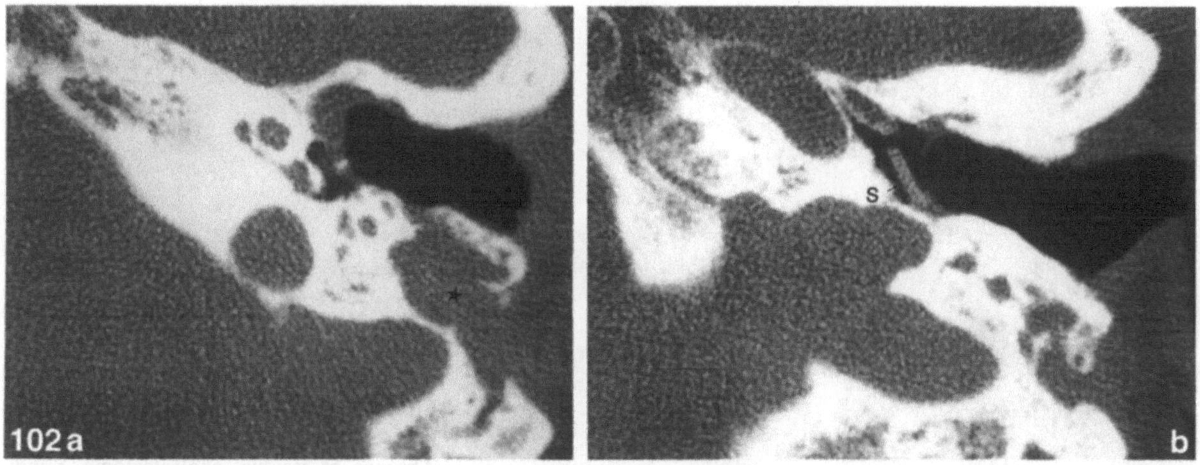

Fig. 102 a,b. High-resolution CT. Horizontal section: partial opacity in tympanic cavity. *s* indicates thick silastic, * complete mastoid opacity: absence of residual cholesteatoma

However, it is interesting to note that none of the patients in our second series required a third operative stage. This has encouraged us to continue using endoscopy, the more so since, from 1990, we have had at our disposal a technique of revision under endoscopic guidance by minimal routes of access, permitting day surgery in over 70% of cases.

CT-endoscopic correlations in the second surgical stage of monitoring closed-technique tympanoplasties

The second, revision, stage in closed techniques for cholesteatoma is virtually routine in our view. But what is the situation with the progress of CT and MRI imaging? Or, in other words, is CT examination adequate for the detection of residual pathology?

According to Voorhees (1983), Oberascher (1989) and Campbell (1990), when there is a free air-filled cavity (fig. 100), high-resolution CT has excellent sensitivity, of the order of 85 to 90%, for the diagnosis of residual cholesteatoma, provided the recurrence exceeds 3 mm in size (fig. 101 a,b).

When partial opacities are present,. it is quite difficult to differentiate between hyperplasia, granulation tissue and a recurrence (figs. 102, 103). For Veillon (1993), hyperplasia is well diagnosed in 92% of cases, likewise fibrosis and a cholesterin-containing granuloma. In difficult cases he opines that CT, combined with MRI, represents an excellent method for detecting the recurrence of a secondary cholesteatoma, previously operated by the closed technique. However, Tono (1989) has shown that, one year after a closed-technique tympanoplasty for cholesteatoma, a CT study on ears presenting a normal tympanum showed that there were only 33% of properly aerated mastoids and 80% of free cavities in the epitympanic region. The difficulty in assessment by CT of residual pathology is further augmented by total opacities of the mastoido-antral cavities due to defective aeration.

In our experience, we have likewise encountered recurrences when the CT was strictly normal (fig. 104). In one case there was a pearl embedded in the round window (fig. 105 a-d), in the other a candle-grease splash of epidermosis of 4 mm applied to the bony auditory meatus opposite the mastoid.

Despite the very good reliability of CT, we continue to perform a second, revision, stage virtually routinely although the use of the endoscope at the first stage, in our experience, has reduced the number of residual cholesteatomas to an eighth. Sometimes the surgeon is unfortunately compelled, for reasons of security in the inner ear, to deliberately leave a little epidermis, as when there is a fistula on a semicrcular canal. A pearl can be observed in a third of cases according to Sanna (1988). It can be removed by endoscopic surgery under video-monitoring.

Sometimes the presence of an epidermosis ensheathing the head of the stapes compels us to leave some epidermal fragments. Residual pathology will then very often be found at the second operative stage of revision. This can then be ablated by the transmeatal route without difficulty.

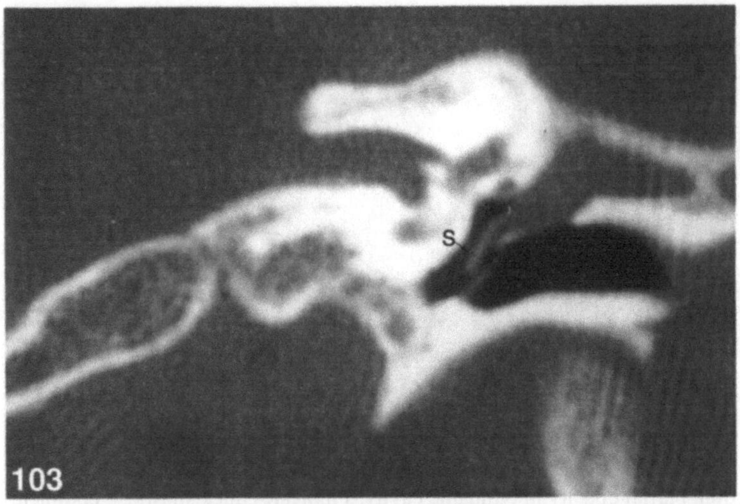

Fig. 103. High-resolution CT. Frontal section: complete opacity of posterior cavities. Absence of residual cholesteatoma. *s* indicates silastic at tympanic cavity

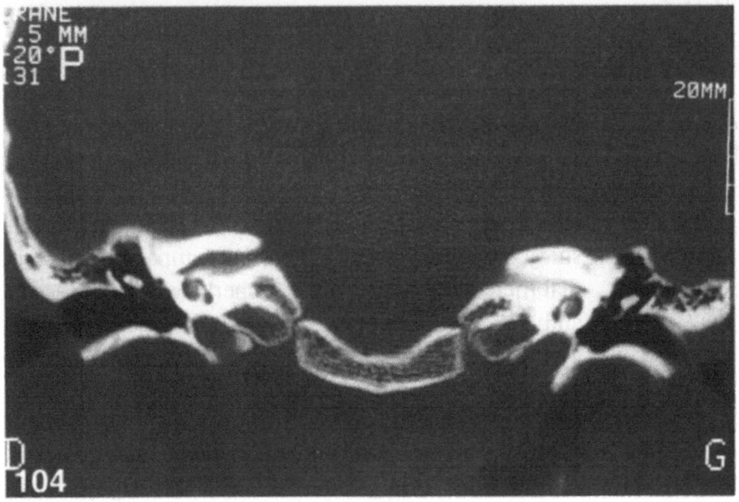

Fig. 104. High-resolution CT. Frontal section: absence of opacity in tympanic cavity; residual cholesteatoma embedded in cochlear niche (cf. fig. 105)

The use of the argon laser (McGee 1983) or the KTP 532 laser (Thedinger 1990) is useful in just such cases to vaporise the epidermal residues atraumatically, likewise to perform ablation of the superstructure of the stapes.

Currently, and for over 70% of our series, we can program revision by endoscopic surgery under day-case conditions. This has the double advantage of reducing the cost of hospitalisation and of being more acceptable to the patient. Such revision allows us not only to eradicate any residual pathology, or to remove the silastic sheet inserted at the first stage to combat the development of fibrosis, but also to improve the hearing if so required by an ossiculoplasty.

Finally, it allows reinforcing surgery for the tympanum in cases with recurrence of a retraction pocket.

References

Campbell J, Pillsbury H (1990) The use of computerized tomographic imaging in revision mastoid surgery for chronic otitis media. Am J Otol 11 : 387-394

Mc Gee T (1983) The argon laser in surgery for chronic ear disease and otosclerosis. Laryngoscope 93 : 1177-1182

Fig. 105 a-h. Right ear: residual cholesteatoma embedded in niche of round window (videoprint). **a** Monitoring of tympanic cavity using 0° optical system: absence of residual pathology; **b, c** epidermal debris at retrotympanic sulcus visible under 70° optical system; **d-f** ablation of residual epidermis under endoscopic guidance; **h** survey at end of eradication: excision satisfactory

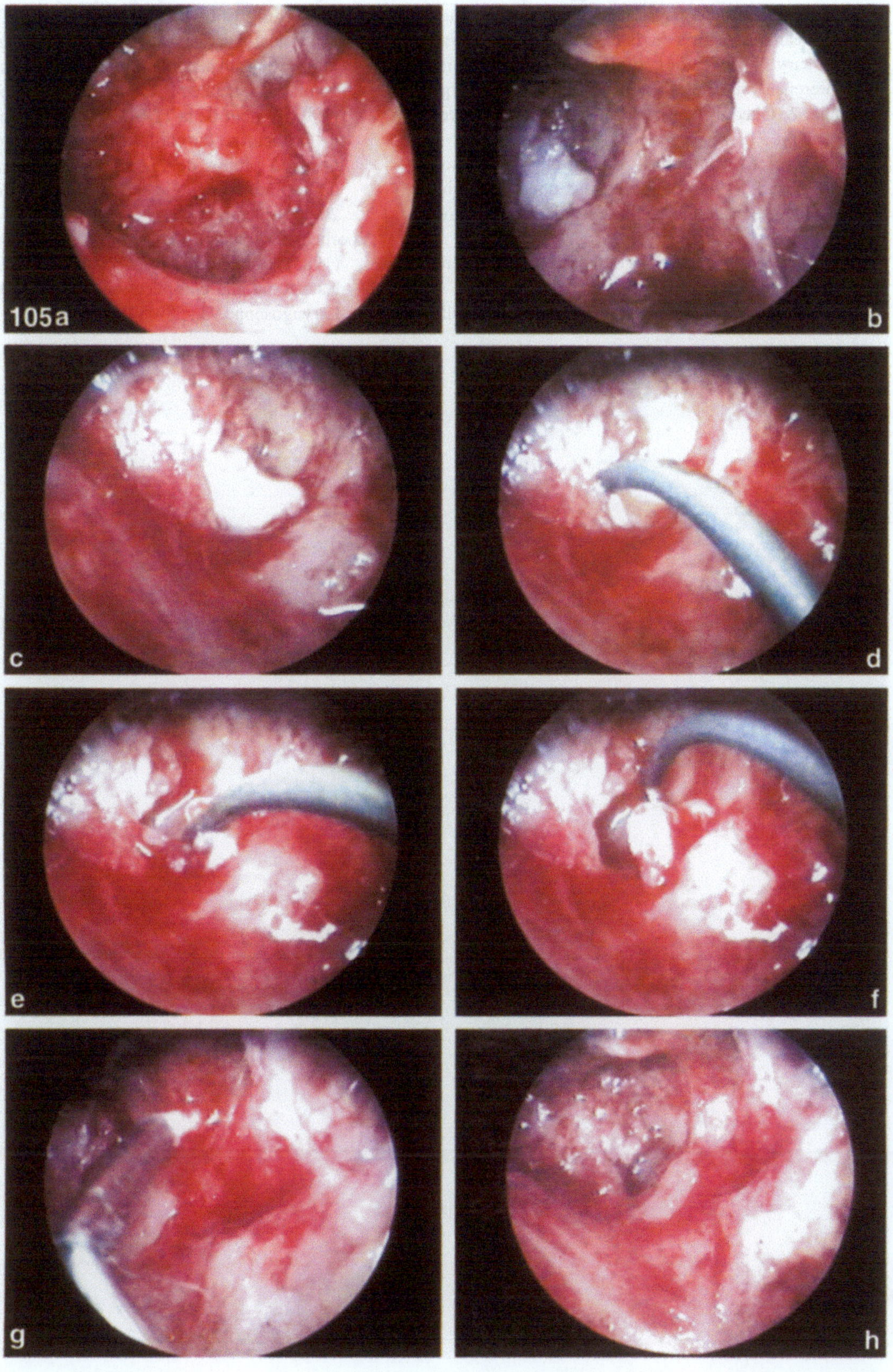
105a
b
c
d
e
f
g
h

Oberascher G, Grobovschek M, Albergger K (1989) The use of high resolution computed tomography to exclude a cholesteatoma recurrence. Is the second-look operation necessary ? Proceeding of the Third International Conference on Cholesteatoma and Mastoid Surgery. Kugler & Ghedini Publications, Amsterdam, Berkeley, Milano pp. 717-720

Sana M, Zini M, Gamoletti R, Taibah A, Russo A, Scandellari R (1988) Closed versus open technique in the management of labyrinthine fistulae. Am J Otol 9 : 470-475

Thedinger B (1990) Applications of the KTP laser in chronic ear surgery. Am J Otol 11 : 79-84

Tono T, Morimitsu T (1989) Postoperative aeration following intact canal wall tympanoplasty evaluation with CT. Proceeding of the Third International Conference on Cholesteatoma and Mastoid Surgery. Kugler & Ghedini Publications, Amsterdam, Berkeley, Milano, pp. 717-720

Veillon F, Le Guennec P, Bourjat P, Conraux C, Stierle JL (1993) Valeur de la TDM et de l'IRM dans la détection de la récidive du cholestéatome de l'oreille moyenne opéré (à propos de 72 cas). 90ème Congrès Français d'Otorhinolaryngolgie et de Pathologie Cervico-faciale, 20-23 septembre

Voorhees R, Johnson D, Lufkin R, Hanafee W, Canalis R (1983) High resolution CT scanning for detection of cholesteatoma and complications in the postoperative ear. Laryngoscope 93 : 589-595

Index

F

H

I, J

L

M

N

O

P

R

MIX
Paper from responsible sources
FSC® C105338

If you have any concerns about our products
you can contact us on
ProductSafety@springernature.com

In case Publisher is established outside the EU,
the EU authorized representative is:
Springer Nature Customer Service Center GmbH
Europaplatz 3, 69115 Heidelberg, Germany

Printed by Libri Plureos GmbH
in Hamburg, Germany

MIX
Papier aus verantwortungsvollen Quellen
Paper from responsible sources
FSC® C105338

If you have any concerns about our products,
you can contact us on
ProductSafety@springernature.com

In case Publisher is established outside the EU,
the EU authorized representative is:
Springer Nature Customer Service Center GmbH
Europaplatz 3, 69115 Heidelberg, Germany

Printed by Libri Plureos GmbH
in Hamburg, Germany